Memoirs Of An Addict:
Fact or Fiction

Memoirs Of An Addict:
Fact or Fiction

M/R Johnson

To: Shanita Burney
Thank you for
your help into
getting the message
of hope to the youth

It is TIME to EDUCATE and ADVOCATE for CHANGE!

Approximately

8.9 million Adults have Co-Occurring Disorders;

7.4 % of individuals receive treatment for both
conditions, while

55.8 % receive no treatment at all.

This book is dedicated to all

who war against

any form of addiction or

mental health disorders or

suicidal ideation

THERE IS HOPE!

DISCLAIMER:

When reading this book if you feel any of the issues herein apply to you personally, you are encouraged to seek an assessment from a qualified Behavioral Health Professional.

To: Memoirs Rhonda Johnson

Through the good times and bad times you have to endure and press on because someone is counting, depending, and trusting in the God in you to lead them out of depression, despair, loneliness, heartache, and worry.

God has place a gift in you that no one else can do or fulfill. In times of questioning, you have to ASK yourself, what is my purpose and will I allow tragedy, death, loss and confusion to stop my assignment from being accomplished?

Grace and Peace,

-Erik Kelley

Order of Content

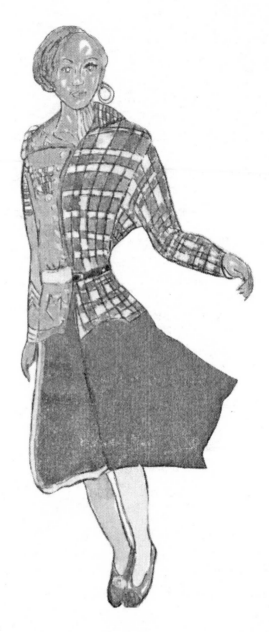

Introducing Mary/Pumpkin

"WORDS CAN BE POWERFUL"

Words can be powerful; carefully put together they are priceless.

What must a caterpillar endure to become a butterfly? The caterpillar's destiny is to survive for the renewing, preparation, and transformation through the metamorphosis stages by reaching the safety of the cocoon. The *purpose* of the process is to receive a reward for the struggle by becoming the beautiful new butterfly creature God intended it to be.

Hello, my name is Mary/Pumpkin; I am one person who has two different personalities and who suffers with a dual diagnosis (co-occurring disorders) of depression and addiction. I happen to be suicidal, yet that is not my story. I am a survivor who lives every day with *hope*. No, life is not always easy and every day is a challenge, but I have learned to become an advocate for change.

Society misuses and misunderstands the word *addict* and needs to understand that everyone has some form of addiction.

It is easy for society to look down on the person suffering with drugs and alcohol, but what about the closet addict who lives every day with an addiction and the world does not see or want to believe they have a problem?

I

I, Mary/Pumpkin, had to learn to examine myself. I had to learn and accept what were the root causes to my addictive, mental, and suicidal behavior.

Once I became a consumer of mental health and received the correct treatment from psychiatric in-patient and outpatient wards along with education from drug rehabilitation programs, my life began to change.

I began to accept my bottom and from there I gained knowledge and took the necessary steps needed to begin my recovery. I learned through recovery how everyone's bottom is not the same and how people with co-occurring disorders battle secret pains and have a story to share.

Most stories shared are the feelings of lost hope, guilt, trauma, low self-esteem, and self-worth, all mixed together with the *shame and stigma* that keeps many enslaved from reaching out for help— this is better known as pride.

The sad part of being an addict was that until I admitted to my addiction and depression, my life had become unmanageable and my process of recovery could not begin.

Once I became true to myself, I accepted the hand of mercy that reached down to save me and I accepted the hand of grace that gave me hope and courage to share my memoirs.

II

Memoirs of An Addict: Fact or Fiction is an extraordinary combined book and workbook that will not save the world, just enlighten and give *hope* that only a Higher Power can save and give any person the necessary tools to defeat addiction, depression, and thoughts of death.

For those who have been blessed and are what the world calls *normal*, I'd like to ask you a question: Can an addict ever be free? Can a person with mental health disorders live a normal life? Or could the answer possibly be in harm reduction?

See, I—Mary/Pumpkin—am a survivor of mental health, drug abuse, and life of suicidal behavior.

For anyone who has walked in my shoes and for those who have not, *Memoirs of An Addict: Fact or Fiction* will give you clarity to why I am no longer among the walking dead.

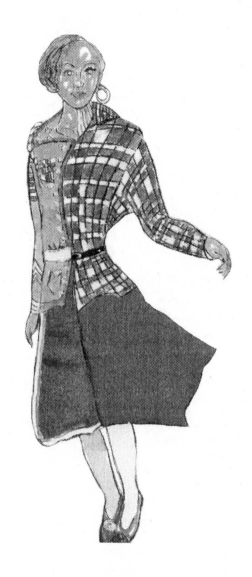

Chapter 1

How It All Began

I'M YOUR DISEASE

I hate meetings. I hate your Higher Power. I hate anyone who has a program. To all who come in contact with me, I wish you death and I wish you suffering.

Allow me to introduce myself. I am the disease of alcoholism and drug addiction. Cunning, baffling, and powerful. That's me. I have killed millions, and I am pleased. I love to catch you with the element of surprise.

I love pretending I am your friend and lover. I have given you comfort, have I not? Wasn't I there? I live to make you hurt. I love to make you cry. Better yet, I love when you are so numb you can neither hurt nor cry. You can't feel anything at all. This is true glory to me.

I will give you instant gratification and all I ask of you is long-term suffering. I've been there for you always. When things were going right in your life, you invited me. You said you didn't deserve these good things, and I was the only one who would agree with you. Together we were able to destroy all things good in your life.

People don't take me seriously. They take strokes seriously, heart attacks seriously, even diabetes they take seriously. Fools that they are, they don't know that without my help these things would not be made possible. I am such a hated disease, and yet I do not come uninvited. You choose to have me. So many have chosen me over reality and peace.

More than you hate me, I hate all of you who have a 12-step program, your programs, your meetings, and your Higher Power. All weaken me and I can't function in the manner I am accustomed to. Now I must lie here quietly. You don't see me, but I am growing bigger than ever. When you only exist, I may live. When you live, I only exist. But I am here…and until we meet again—if we meet again—I wish you death and suffering. I am your disease.

– Author unknown

Mary, you are so beautiful, why you are using drugs? What happened in your life to make you an addict? What's wrong, Mary? Can you tell me why you like getting high?

Well, since you asked me what's going on I will try to explain. I'm depressed, I'm hurting, I'm hearing voices, I'm lost, and I need to know—can someone help me before it's too late? I find the only thing that keeps me in my right mind is having someone to let me know I'm not alone in how I'm feeling.

Being depressed is like living in a black hole. There is no light in sight, just voices trying to point me the way out. Some good and some bad. So please, someone tell me or explain to me what's really going on? Why do you see the outside of me, yet you fail to see what's going on inside of me?

All I want is help not to feel this way. All I want is a chance to be what the world calls normal. Yes, I'm an addict but that's not my story.

Now before you make up your mind to judge me and my addiction, how about you get to know me first.

I am a native Washingtonian raised in a two-parent home. My family is old school, meaning family comes first. My family understood the importance of family traditions and the value of knowing and trusting in God. I was raised believing you are nothing if you don't have family. My family would meet on Sundays for dinner and every holiday was the highlight of my childhood. My mama would say protect, love, and watch each other, for the family is the heart of survival.

I grew up near the Washington Navy Yard and near the Washington Wharf in SW Washington, DC. The part of SW I claim is P Street.

My neighborhood was made of mixed races and creeds of people. There were poor people as well as people of stature (celebrities, as well as politicians)—yes, I grew up around people with money.

I am so glad my parents afforded me the opportunity to learn diversity early in my childhood.

I never know there was a separation between black and white people as a child. I learned early to be careful how you treat people; you never know who you might need in this life, for to tell the truth we all bleed the same.

I was eight years old, a tiny little skinny statuesque girl with more legs than body. My eyes were a stunning brown that radiated as if I was able to see through a person's soul and be able to discern the type of character they possessed. Really, I was a child before my time, an old spirit that was trapped in a young girl's body. I feared no one and, keeping it real, I was the one to fear. Confidence was not my problem although as a child I walked as if I owned the world.

Yet, I had issues: I was depressed and I needed someone to enlighten me as to why my voices were telling me to hurt myself.

I was too young to handle what was transpiring in my life. There were unexplainable entities and visions that I as a little girl experienced, and regular doctors, teachers, and family members were amazed and could not believe a child so young could have insight of events before my time.

I had a creative mind and enjoyed talking to myself. Maybe it was my creativity that helped me cope with my undiagnosed mental illness.

I enjoyed talking to myself out loud as if there was someone near me having a conversation.

I remember how my mama would always tell me, "Mary stop talking to yourself" as if it was not normal, speaking to those voices that kept telling me to hurt myself. Maybe what I was hearing was my imagination gone wild.

Growing up, I would meet with a special friend that only I could talk to. We arranged a meeting place where we would not be interrupted and only we knew this place existed. It was our place of peace.

It was not too far from my home, so I could travel alone and not be in harm's danger of child predators.

All my concentration was on just reaching my place of peace so I could talk to my voices and speak freely to them while having my special date with my friend who I called me, myself, and I.

We would meet as often as possible on a little street that was closed off, so no cars could travel on it. It was made of several wide white-square bricks that were used as the sidewalks. This little closed-off street housed high-rise apartments as well.

There you could see families walking dogs and riding their bikes. You could hear the laugher of human voices as they were enjoying the beauty of the scenic environment.

For me the sidewalk reminded me of white sand that would lead me to my personal beach.

I would give the white brick path a name that I called my wide brick road, and every time I traveled to my place of peace I thought I was Dorothy from *The Wizard of Oz*.

I would sing the "Yellow Brick Road" song in the heat or in the rain; I would sing in the cold or in the snow to follow the wide brick road, follow, follow, and follow the wide brick road until I would reach the ocean.

Yes, that's correct—I said the ocean. I had a personal ocean living in SW Washington, DC. It is known as the Anacostia River. It was dirty—full of trash, empty bottles, and dead fish floating. Sometimes the smell of the dead fish would be so bad that a person could have gotten sick.

For a child before my time, I was able to use my creative mind in the midst of the trash and pollutions the river possessed.

To me, the river was beautiful and it was my ocean like no other ocean in the world. You could see the airplanes leaving from Washington National Airport. You could see the cars traveling on the streets from East Potomac Park known as Haines Point, while watching the boats ride up and down the river.

I could see the beauty in between the dirty trash bags. I could see the beauty in each bottle that floated with every wave going back and forth as if I was traveling with each bottle looking to reach a destination.

I could see the beauty in all the dead fish that were beating against this long white wall that housed the police water patrol. I gave the wall the name *It's The End of the Road.* I liked that name; it seemed suitable for all the dead smelly fish that had nowhere else to go.

But no matter to me. Every day I followed my white wide brick road and I would meet me, myself, and I as often as I could. I never wanted to leave but I had to go home.

While at home I would talk to myself about what great a day I had.

To prevent my family from saying, "Here she goes again, talking to herself," I would just wait for my scheduled date to speak to my special friend and tell me, myself, and I that I made it through another day without trying to kill myself.

My mama knew something was wrong with me. I would hear her say to my daddy, "I think your daughter has a mental problem." Being the middle child of three and trying to find my place in the family, maybe I suffered the middle child syndrome and did not know where I fitted in. All I can remember was being depressed, and to make things worse, I would cry a lot.

Looking back, people said I acted the way I did for attention; my mama knew that was not the case because I stayed under her like flies on honey. She couldn't even go to the bathroom in peace without me hanging on her legs.

I loved my mama and daddy so much. Yet, I was Mama and Daddy's problem child.

I gave my mama hell and all she wanted me to do was stop crying and talk to a doctor, a psychiatrist to see what was wrong with her little girl.

My mama would make pediatric appointments to see if I was sick with something, only to be informed psychically nothing was wrong with me.

When Mama suggested to my daddy that I see a psychiatrist, my daddy said no. My daddy said he was not going to have his little girl talking to a psychiatrist and being stigmatized as someone with a mental illness. This was not heard of or accepted in the African American community.

The only time people in the African American community went to see a psychiatrist; they had some kind of physical disability. The people with mental illnesses went to Saint Elizabeth Hospital here in Washington, DC. Only God knows what type of treatment or medication and care a black child received from an asylum hospital. Black children in those places had no rights.

Before you judge my mama and daddy, Google and read the information concerning mental hospitals for children before 1980.

My daddy believed I was spoiled, not crazy. See, I was Daddy's little girl. My daddy worked two jobs to take care of his family and because my daddy worked so much, he never got to see me in my raw or out-bursting form, as if I was a psycho child from hell.

My daddy was my world and I knew he loved me unconditionally. He stood up for me and he would always talk and encouraged me not to cry. One Christmas, my daddy gave me this baby doll. He whispered in my ear "I love you" and "Now you have someone you can talk to."

This doll was as big as I was. She was so beautiful with long hair with which I could create a new hairstyle every day. She always wore a smile and gave me love. I called her Suzy. I loved Suzy so much; she was my best friend when I could not get outside to see me, myself, and I.

I would tell Suzy everything and she would listen. I would tell her I was about to kill myself and all she did was listen. She never judged me. We would have tea parties and dress up events. She was all I had that understood me.

See, Suzy loved me and it did not matter how bad I felt; she would always listen. When I felt alone and just wanted to run away, Suzy was there. She would always tell me that it was going to be okay. She was the best thing in my life and besides my daddy, I believed only Suzy loved me.

She would always tell me to stop crying, don't kill yourself, everything is going to be alright.

I don't know; maybe I cried a lot because my mama cried a lot when she was pregnant with me. She was only fourteen when she had her first child and then she was pregnant with me at fifteen.

Maybe it was the stress she was experiencing at the time before my birth that created this sense of hopelessness.

Once my daddy's family found out she was pregnant again with me, my parents were told they had to get married. Maybe she was not ready for all that. Maybe that's why my mama cried while pregnant and it just rubbed off on me.

See, I know my mama loved me, even though I cried for hours and hours. You tell me what parent could handle a child under those situations and not think something was wrong with their child.

It's not my mama's fault; maybe I loved her too much and required too much of her time. Maybe she was angry with me because she had to get married so young and stay at home to take care of her children at such a young age. I don't know and I don't have a true answer.

I don't think my mama ever looked at being pregnant with me as a blessing. Hell, it wasn't easy for my daddy either; he was only seventeen years old; a real man who stood up and accepted his responsibilities. I loved them both so much. They were truly parents from God, examples that love and marriage can work, for they were married for forty years until death did them part.

All I know is no one could see my pain or understand I was hearing voices and how I was suffering within.

They say knowledge is power and every family has a secret. Little did my family know mental health disorders of depression and bipolar disorder run in the family. It was not until the death of my grandma when the truth was finally told.

If only the family was educated that mental health disorders can be passed down just like bad eyes or diabetes or cancer from generation to generation.

Maybe it was the shame and stigma of mental health disorders why I and children of my generation did not get the correct treatment.

As a child, most of the time I wished I were dead. I just wanted to die and be away from the voices and the pain. I remember asking myself what was my purpose for being here on this planet. I hated myself and I hated being around people except Suzy.

ATTENTION! ATTENTION!

When you see or hear of stories such as this, know and understand this is a sure sign of depression and something is wrong. No child cries for hours and hours and no child should say over and over I wish I were dead. *This is a cry for help!*

My mama was right: something was wrong with me. I should have got help early. Maybe I would not be an addict now. The reality of becoming an addict: Tragedy had to happen in my life before I ever got help. So many suffering addicts are crying for professional therapy—and they need help.

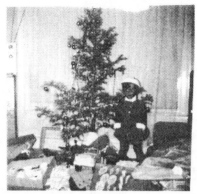

Suzy

The National Institute for Mental Health released an article concerning depression and other disorders at their website: www.nimh.nih.gov/health/topics/depression.

Major depressive disorder can be described as feeling sad, blue, unhappy, miserable, or down in the dumps. Most of us feel this way at one time or another for short periods. Depression can change or distort the way you see yourself, your life, and those around you. True clinical depression is a mood disorder in which feelings of sadness, loss, anger, or frustration interfere with everyday life for weeks or longer. Depression can change or distort the way you see yourself, your life, and those around you.

The exact cause of depression is not known. Many researchers believe it is caused by chemical changes in the brain. This may be due to a problem with your genes, or it can be triggered by certain stressful events. More likely, it's a combination of both. Some types of depression run in families, but

17

depression can also occur if you have no family history of the illness. Anyone can develop depression—even kids—or even alcohol or drug abuse can play a role in depression.

Certain medical conditions that include underactive thyroid, cancer, or long-term pain, or even some medications such as steroids can cause depression.

Sleeping problems or stressful life events such as breaking up with a boyfriend or girlfriend, failing a class, or the death or illness of someone close to you are also strong factors in causing depression.

People who have been divorced, have suffered childhood abuse or neglect, have lost their jobs, or face social isolation (common in the elderly) are more at risk for developing depression.

People who suffer from depression usually see everything with a more negative attitude. They cannot imagine that any problem or situation can be solved in a positive way.

Symptoms of depression can include agitation, restlessness, and irritability. A person can be withdrawn or isolated and have difficulty concentrating or may notice a dramatic change in appetite, often resulting in weight gain or loss. People can experience fatigue and lack of energy, feelings of hopelessness and helplessness as well as feelings of worthlessness, self-hate, and guilt.

In my own depression journey, I lost interest or pleasure in activities that I once enjoyed. I suffered thoughts of death or suicide, and experienced trouble sleeping or slept too much.

Reading and realizing I experienced these symptoms of depression was a wake-up call. It is important for people to understand that depression can also appear as anger and discouragement rather than feelings of sadness that most people associate depression with.

If depression is very severe, there may also be psychotic symptoms, such as hallucinations and delusions. In these cases or if an individual with depression is suicidal or extremely depressed and cannot function, they may need to be treated in a psychiatric hospital.

People who are depressed are more likely to use alcohol or illegal substances. Complications of depression also include increased risk of health problems, such as suicide.

A person who has thoughts of hurting themselves or committing suicide should call a doctor right away. Other symptoms including hearing voices that are not there or having frequent crying spells with little or no reason that is disrupting work, school, or family life should warrant an immediate trip to the doctor.

TELL SOMEONE PLEASE!

Just think—if I would have been successful in hurting and killing myself I would not be able to share this message that there is *hope*!

Fast forward. I am now thirteen years old. My poor Suzy…I have cut her hair, painted her nails, and put on lipstick. I have messed up my poor friend. No matter what I did to beautify Suzy, she always told me I would always have her until the end. Just like a true friend.

I stopped meeting my special friend—me, myself, and I—after Suzy came into my life to become my best friend. But from time to time I still would travel there to my place of peace because I loved being among the earth.

One day while at my place of peace, I met an acquaintance. He was one of the neighborhood thugs—a little older than me. He would always say he liked my style of being straightforward with the things I would say.

For me, that was a compliment because I had a smart mouth. My mama would say, "You are too grown" and she would have me wash my mouth out with soap. Mama knew beating or spanking me did not work. (I had got to the point that when I was being spanked I would travel inside my mind and be somewhere else. After a while, my mama knew spanking me didn't work. However, washing my mouth out with the soap did.)

The neighborhood thug asked if I wanted to try his funny cigarette. He explained to me that it was called a joint—in short, it was marijuana. I said okay.

Wow! My first experience was like the movie *Half Baked*—man, I could not stop laughing. We hung out together until I came down from the high. For the first time my brain experienced something that calmed those voices and racing thoughts. This marijuana—good, bad, right, or indifferent—became my medication at just thirteen years of age.

For those who are unaware, marijuana is the gateway to the devil's pit of addiction. Yes, for my young friends marijuana comes from the earth but it comes with a price and it is called *addiction*.

Now you might ask: Mary, how were you able to buy marijuana at such an early age?

Well, you know how the saying goes: it's not what you know; it's how you use what you know. I never used my body or sold my soul to the devil. Every time I got the marijuana, those voices were calm—which calmed me.

This is when I started by life as a closet addict. I didn't want anyone in my family to know I was getting high.

One day after hanging out with my thug friend, my mama and daddy asked to speak to me. *Man*, I thought to myself, *I'm in trouble. They know I'm getting high.* But little did I know what they wanted to speak to me was much more intense than that.

Daddy and Mama asked me to come into their room. My little legs began to shake and I began to sweat as if I was guilty and had to expose that I had been smoking marijuana. I slowly walked into my parents' room trying not to look guilty.

My parents didn't waste any time with what they had to tell me.

"Mary, we need you to tell Suzy goodbye."

Now I'm stunned because they know how important she is to me.

"What do you mean tell Suzy goodbye, Mama?"

With tears running down my face and with anger in my voice I ask, "WHY! What did I do wrong? I'll take better care of her, I promise!"

21

I sat between Mama and Daddy crying, for the weed had worn off and I was not ready for this type of drama.

"But Daddy, please! Suzy is my best friend and I need her."

"No, Mary, we are moving to Maryland and Suzy cannot come," he said as he wiped away my tears.

I was relieved—I wasn't in trouble for smoking marijuana. Now feeling the downside of the drug, I began to shout: "I don't want to move! I like it here, Daddy."

"Well, baby, we are moving this Friday."

How do I say goodbye to Suzy? How do I say goodbye to my best friend?

This experience jolted me to the core. I was no longer me—I became Mary.

With her head held down and tears in her eyes, Mary walked into her room to prepare to talk to Suzy. She began to prepare their last dinner party together with all the stuff animals she could find.

It would not be easy for Mary to say goodbye, so she prepared a speech for Suzy and the guests.

"Suzy," Mary began, "you have been my best friend and I will never forget you. You have been more than my doll baby and I love you but I cannot take you with me to my new home. Mama and Daddy said you cannot go."

Then Mary broke out and shouted, "I am so sorry, Suzy! Thank you for being there for me. Thank you for always listening to me. I am so sorry I can't take you with me."

She wiped the tears from her face and told Suzy again how much she loved her and how important she had been to her life.

As Mary moved away from the table, she called her daddy to the room and he took Suzy away. Until this day I don't know what Daddy did with her…all I knew was my best friend Suzy was gone.

Suzy was just a doll baby, but giving up Suzy was like a baby having to give up its pacifier. It was equivalent of having to give up that comfort blanket or a favorite stuffed animal like a teddy bear or that favorite shirt or dress.

It's Friday, moving day. The family lineage from Washington DC is being transported to Maryland.

Maryland was nothing like living in DC. It was a whole new world for Mary. She was by herself with no place of peace, no Suzy, and no weed to smoke.

Since Mary had always been an introvert, being by herself was okay, but she was bored.

Her family had moved to a town called Forestville. There were trees…and trees…and more tress up and down the highway.

For Mary, living Maryland was nice, but there was no ocean or place of peace she could visit. The poor kids she met were just not cool enough nor were they on the same page as Mary.

At her new school, the kids had old souls— they were Maryland kids who knew little about DC. All the new girls she would meet were the same age and none of them smoked cigarettes or marijuana.

Mary would call them little goody goody's girls because they didn't even drink beer.

I got to get out of here. I got to get to DC to get me some weed, Mary thought to herself again and again.

Every weekend, Mary tried to find a way to get to her grandma's house, who lived in southeast Washington, DC. It was about eleven, maybe thirteen miles to walk. Mary had to learn the route because the Maryland bus transportation system stopped bus services early and she didn't want to be stuck in Maryland on the weekends.

Mary knew people who lived around her grandma's house that she could hang with and possibly get her marijuana from.

Mary and her grandma had a special relationship. Grandma was the matriarch—the nuts and bolts that built the foundation of the family. She was beautiful and loving and had a spirit of God that understood Mary better than anyone in the family. Grandma knew how to calm Mary down when she was having her little fits. Oh yeah! Grandma believed in talking, but she had a whip to let you know she wasn't playing.

Grandma would tell Mary stories of her life— the good times and bad times when life was hard for her raising kids alone because Mary's grandfather died at an early age. Grandma said that no matter how many challenges she had, the LORD had always brought her through.

Mary would tell Grandma almost everything except her smoking marijuana. She would share with Grandma concerning her voices and tell her how people, family, and friends would laugh at her for having skinny legs.

Grandma would encourage Mary with words of wisdom by instructing her to pray for those people and not to get mad or upset when people started talking about her. "Always remember there are people who don't have legs at all, so be thankful for the little skinny legs you have," Grandma would say. Grandma always knew how to make the negative into a positive.

Grandma believed in the power of prayer and she believed in teaching the family to exercise the power of prayer to know God for themselves.

She would always tell Mary to be prepared, for a day was coming in her life that trouble would surround her and danger would be in her face. Grandma would always stress, "Mary, you must believe and know for yourself that God can do anything but fail."

Their relationship was greater than that of an average grandmother and granddaughter, for Mary was being educated concerning the principalities and rulers of darkness. Grandma would teach Mary by reinforcing the scriptures. In order for Mary to go outside, she had to learn and know the Lord's Prayer and Psalm 23.

Although Mary had a motive for coming to DC, she never smoked any marijuana while she was at Grandma's house, but she did find a way to take a joint home.

It's now the mid 1980s—Mary is in her teens and she is preparing to start high school. Mary is smoking marijuana every day and is still getting high by herself like a junkie or weed head keeping their addiction a secret. Only occasionally she would meet up with some of her marijuana buddies to smoke a joint before school—most of the time, she enjoyed getting high by herself.

One day while sitting on the wall at her high school, a classmate named John was playing his music box with this crazy new beat.

"What's that music you're listening to?" Mary asked. "I've never heard that beat before. It's funky!"

John turned the music up louder and told her it was called go-go and the song playing was called "Bustin' Loose" by Chuck Brown and the Soul Searcher.

He pulled out a joint and Mary and John partied until they went to class singing "I feel like bustin' loose."

John would tell Mary about an event where Chuck Brown and other go-go bands would be playing for the weekend. For Mary, this was the beginning of an era where she would fit in with party people who loved the go-go music of Washington, DC.

Go-go music was a mixture of blues, funk, and hip-hop blended together. Each band represented a different sound and flavor. Mary loved everything about it. There were all-night go-go spots like the Howard Theater, the Monistic Temple, the Celebrity Hall, and other spots where the young people could meet and enjoy being young.

Every weekend there was something to do. This new and exciting era also brought a new magnitude of drugs and getting high. No longer was marijuana the thing or the drug to do. No! A new drug called Love Boat or PCP was the choice drug now.

Man, people were jumping off buildings and acting like they had super strength as if they were cursed with some form of a demon in their bodies. It was crazy—and Mary was smoking those crazy drugs as well.

Stop—before I go any further I have to inform you what ingredients made up the drug Love Boat.

A. You needed marijuana to lace the drug-- *Excuse me,* I mean to *place on top* of the marijuana.

B. One of the drug's main ingredients is embalming fluid.

Yes, that's right—people in Washington, DC were smoking the chemical that the funeral morgue used in dead people's bodies. The drug was like the drug Angel Dust—and Mary smoked and loved every minute of it.

Before you judge Mary smoking Love Boat, pull out that which is in your eye first.

This is what addiction does. It makes you lose your mind by sniffing glue or paint, or shooting heroin in your veins or smoking a blunt or drinking cough syrup with soda, or smoking K2…and yes, even ingesting dead people's embalming fluid to smoke PCP.

It is now the late 1980s and it is summertime in Washington, DC. Mary is home watching the news on the television and getting ready to meet up with some people who are going to see the go-go bands EU and Rare Essence at the Howard Theater later that night.

The news anchor on the television is saying, "We are interrupting our regular television programming for a breaking story."

The breaking story was concerning a new drug that had hit New York City.

The news anchor spoke and looked into the camera as if he had seen death.

"Good evening. A new drug called crack has hit New York City with a vengeance. This new drug is a form of cocaine with a highly addictive taste."

He warned the listening audience that once a person indulges in this new drug called crack, they would be instantly addicted.

He presented a series of images of people who were leaving their place of employment for lunch to purchase the drug crack and going into abandoned buildings to smoke it. The term, he stated, was called freebasing.

He showed images of people using different types of glass pipes, aluminum cans, or whatever worked to smoke their new drug.

He also reported that this drug was affecting people on all walks of life from the rich to the poor.

Some people were selling their bodies and their babies to get this new drug.

He stressed to the listening audience as if a hurricane was about to hit land to start preparing for this new drug called crack, as it was coming to their city and towns.

Mary was not impressed by the breaking news story so she continued to get dressed.

Oh my gosh! What is this man talking about? People in DC are too busy hanging at the go-go and smoking PCP to be a part of that madness.

Little did Mary know this new drug called crack cocaine—the devil's drug—would change the course of history.

America would never be the same. It was like an inside plot of terrorism to destroy the make-up of American families and create a new way of living.

In Mary's mind, this news was depressing. All she could think about was getting high on the Love Boat, so out the door she went.

Later that evening Mary met up with her Love Boat buddies.

"Hey, what's up, people? How are ya living? Ready to go in and party?"

"Girl! You won't believe this—we have been looking all day for the Love Boat."

"What do you mean all day? Did ya get it?"

"No! We couldn't find it anywhere."

It was as if Mary had been hit by a train. "No! This can't happen." With no PCP, Mary looked like she had lost her best friend.

All she kept thinking in the back of her mind was the breaking news stories about the new drug called crack. She wondered if this was the reason

29

why there was no Love Boat and if this was the beginning before the storm.

"Well does anybody have some weed?" she asked, desperate.

"Girl! Marijuana is in demand right now! If we could have got our hands on some weed we would have big money in our pockets right now."

"Then what are we going to do?"

"I'm ready to float on the water with no Love Boat to carry me. Maybe somebody will have some drugs when we get inside."

Mary went into the Howard Theater with no luck of finding any marijuana or Love Boat at all.

Crack cocaine was the only drug available, so Mary started smoking crack. From time to time Mary did drink alcohol and beer but her body was addicted to smoking drugs and her mind and body was used to a certain type of escapism.

This new drug crack made people different. This drug turned straight men gay and turned women away from their homes. Prostitution had nothing on the crack whores, for they would sell their bodies for two bucks just to get a hit.

The thing to smoking crack—you did not go outside except to buy more drugs.

Crack made you the devil's prisoner by making it affordable. Once a person smoked crack, you wanted more and more and more.

To this day you can never get enough. It always seemed like when people got their first good hit from the drug, most of the time the money was gone.

There is a quote that states, "One is too many and a thousand is never enough."

I would not wish that addiction on my worst enemy. Yet, people Mary loved—family and friends—became out of control addicts too. No one escaped crack, and Mary became a prisoner as well.

With the drug crack it didn't matter if you were rich or poor. When you smoked crack, you became a slave of the devil.

So should I lie and tell you if Mary never touched marijuana or smoked Love Boat she would not be addicted to crack now? Or should I lie and say crack cocaine just happened by mistake or by *accident?*

The fact is drugs are the downfall for people who have issues that need to be addressed. Crack just became a source for the enemy to start building a kingdom for bondage so you could be a slave to addiction.

Crack cocaine became an epidemic and not even President George Bush Sr. had answers how to stop the devastation.

People were becoming depressed without answers, never realizing the truth to what was really happening, that a beast from the eternal pit of Hell and his demons had arrived on Earth.

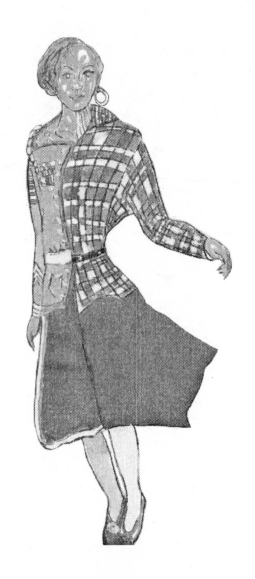

Chapter 2

Stories of the Dungeon

Oh my God! What was that loud thundering noise? Why are people taking cover? I hear something...

Fffffsssssffffffs...BOOOOOOOM!

The S bomb of mass destruction has just exploded. Strong, propagating shock waves travel outward in a white powder mushroom cloud that appears to be releasing some form of contamination of lethal poison.

A great ball of fire where the S bomb has landed has cracked the earth. The force of the fire is reaching toward the sky. I don't know for sure, but in the mist of the fire, rays appear to be images of witches on their brooms, ghosts, and some form of soldiers with wide tails and wings on their backs; they are marching out of the fire into the atmosphere.

The white powder funnel cloud is heading toward New York City, Detroit, Colorado, California, and Washington, DC.

The TNT in the S bomb, better known as Satin's Bomb, contains crack cocaine triggering a nation of crack zombies.

The death toll and devastation is unknown. Fallout shelters have become dungeons for the legions of villainous demon solders to set up their

33

kingdom of crack houses. It appears no city or state is safe from this new epidemic.

"May God be with us" was all Mary could say, for she was an addict who did not escape the attack and she could see firsthand the havoc crack was having in Washington DC, a city that would become known as the murder capital of the world.

It is now the late 80s and early 90s. Crack cocaine has changed the way of life. This immoral monster, crack the rock, was taking over and no one seemed to have answers how to stop the impact of the devastation.

A new sheriff has come to town—an overseer whose main purpose was to implement the devil's plan by releasing the seven deadly sins into existence—the sins of lust, gluttony, greed, laziness, wrath, envy, and pride.

This new sheriff sought devious, monstrous, vicious, and murderous souls who were willing to do the devil's business through crack cocaine.

The dungeon became the central point and haven place for the lost souls whose spirits were prisoners to their addiction to crack, for in the dungeon you could find shelter, drugs, detestable sins, or sexual pleasure from men and women while hanging with Satan himself.

Those who became victims usually had low self-esteem, infirmities, turmoil, and were not able to deal with the shame from being addicted to crack.

Those victims who had one foot in the dungeon and one foot with the church were not allowed to break the cycle because they lived in denial, so for many who would say "I would never smoke crack" became crack heads lost from pride and became hopeless because crack took them to places they should have never gone.

The dungeon was the devil's playground and those with a strong dependence to crack were more often treated like unclean lepers who lived in bondage and would inflict physical and emotional pain on each other.

The life of the dungeon would be the place of excuses to use drugs.

It doesn't matter what form of addiction a person has; upon entering into the dungeon, a person has a place to run to and escape reality by running from *themself.*

You couldn't find one addict who wanted to admit they had an addiction, or admit they were powerless.

"Beam me up, Scotty" was the slogan. People were selling their souls just to go into a fantasy world called space to reach the enterprise known as the gates of hell.

What made crack so dangerous was several factors: the low cost, how easy it was to manufacture the drug, and the profits.

I tell you greed and envy was running neck to neck. But let's not forget gluttony, for anyone addicted to crack could tell you once you hit the crack rock, you could never get enough.

The devil made the drug crack look like candy and any person could buy the drug with as little as five dollars from the neighborhood drug dealer.

Not only were people addicted to crack in DC, but also people of all colors, race, and creed were coming from Virginia and Maryland to DC to purchase the drug as well.

The high lasted about five to fifteen minutes. It would rush to the brain quickly as if it was the highest climax one could get while having sex. The smoke looked and flowed from the pipe as if it was the cum of the devil's penis.

The best way to describe the excitement of the high was like a person who loves to eat crabs. I don't care how much butter you have or that special sauce you fix or how many crabs you crack to eat, you just can't seem to get full enough...so you tend to eat more and more and more. Why? Because the sensation of cracking the crabs has become tireless and the need for the meat is over.

Now with crack cocaine you never get tired; you just want more and more knowing after that first hit you would not get the same sensations. That is when most of the time the money would run out first.

It has been said that only the drug heroin takes the body through serious withdrawals.

Man that is a lie! Let Mary tell you differently.

Crack takes the body, mind, and spirit through withdrawals as well. During the evolution era of crack, people had the symptoms of depression from the lack of money, fatigue from the lack of sleep, anxiety that caused tremors that made one irritable, and mental cravings for more and more of the drug.

Withdrawals from crack is real, not fiction. This is fact from a person who lived and experienced firsthand what her body went through.

During the 90s, crack had people killing, stealing, and destroying themselves and others to get that hit of escapism. That is what made the dungeon the haven and the devil's playground.

As long as you were willing to do the devil's business, your addiction was going to be fed.

Stories of the dungeon and the life of crack gave true meaning to the saying: be careful how you treat people; you never know who you might need; you never know who would be the one to help you or give you your last cup of water, or who will be there when you are sick, without any money, down in spirit, and have lost hope.

Listen! Be quiet! Turn the lights off! No, wait, look out the windows; I hear something…I think it is the police! Mary is all alone hiding in her closet. She is high from smoking crack and she is paranoid.

A closet addict enslaved by her addiction. She is smoking, drinking, and seeking temporary pleasure. Trying to escape her problems by not facing the crack demon has become her god.

But who is Mary running from when no one is there but her and her crack pipe? Maybe she is hiding in the closet so God the Father and her family won't see how crack has turned her into a living walking dead zombie.

Mary the closet addict's body and mind has become dependent on the effects of the drug. Smoking crack has become a normal way of life and to make matters worse, she is the worst type of addict—she likes to get high by herself.

Mary would say getting high by herself would cause less confusion and she could smoke and spend her money at a pace where she would always have something at the end of the high.

Mary had a small circle of associates who were crack smokers and she could feel comfortable smoking with them. Most of them were trying to hide and keep their addiction under the table. Few people knew of her addiction.

The devil knew he had Mary, for as long as she was a closet addict who did not want her family to know she smoked crack, she would always be a slave.

One day, Mary was walking down the street with no money feeling sick while having an anxiety attack. Thoughts of death were entering into her mind. She was sad and depressed; all she wanted to do was get high. Mary was hurting. It seemed like that the devil was talking to her saying, "Just take some money from your family; they will never know."

Yeah right!

Mary at that time was not willing to take that chance.

It has been said that a person addicted to crack will sell their body to feed their addiction. That's not always true. It's sad how that stigma about people—especially women—and their addiction to drugs work.

Some women did not have to sell their bodies because women like closet addict Mary would use their brains. Let's call it manipulation.

Truth be told, not all women in addiction sell their bodies all that time. Let's talk…. More straight men sell their integrity to get high on crack, creating the down-low experience. This is one of the main reasons men brought sexually transmitted diseases home to the women that help create HIV and AIDS.

Mary never had a problem. As long as she had ten bucks, she could work some type of magic. She could monitor her addiction by getting high by herself. See, that's the only thing that saved her; she was a closet addict.

Mary was sick in her addiction. She needed help because she was a prisoner a closet addict trapped by crack. It didn't matter how much marijuana or Love Boat she smoked. Crack was different—it could make a person feel relaxed then it could make you feel dirty.

For the non-closet addicts, this is how people spent their whole paycheck, got lost, and messed up their families hanging at the dungeon.

Some people did not like smoking crack by themselves, which made them prey or weak soul candidates known as suckers, so they had to pay and take the abuse of the predators who made them spend all their money on drugs and they never got high for all the money they spent.

For those who wonder why their mates never had money, the devil really assisted the cause. First you had to pay the house to enter into the dungeons to smoke the drugs. Then you had to pay a runner to go get the drug. Now you had to pay to use the crack pipe. Next you had to pay to use the lighter. Then you had to pay so the person would leave you alone so you could smoke your crack for just one minute in peace. Next you had to find a cigarette. Before you knew it, time had passed and it's now five o'clock in the morning and all the money from your paycheck is gone.

Now you are so geeked out and paranoid that the person you paid to stay in the dungeon is putting you out of the house so you have to spend more money to stay so you can get yourself together. By the time the sun is shining, you are broke with no money, no cigarettes, and no lighter, and are trying to figure out how you are going to pay your bills when you just got paid.

Crack has its own entities like no other drug. Because the drug high is so short lived it is one of the most dangerous drugs to man. It talks to you like a person and it totally takes over. It could make you lose your mind by bringing all your fears into existence.

During all the madness of the crack era, Mary's mama told her if she or anyone in the family smoked that devil's d*** she would disown them.

On another day Mary could not work her ten-dollar magic, for she had no money and she wanted to get high. The closet addict, with nowhere to go, walking with her head down to the ground as if she was looking for a crack rock, found a dollar.

WOW! I need this dollar, Mary said as she headed toward the neighborhood convenience store to buy a beer and calm her nerves.

Mary walked into the store and opened the glass case where all the beers were housed, knowing she better purchase the right beer. The winner of the dollar was Steele Reserved 211.

Man, it's a sad thing to be a closet addict and have no money, no cigarettes, no lighter, no drugs, and no place to go to get high for free when you are down on your luck.

That was all Mary was thinking about as she was leaving the store.

Happy to have been able to buy the cheap beer, she walked out the store to hear a strong voice saying, "Put your head up; there is nothing on the ground!"

She looked up to see a tall thin man who looked like he had just finished painting a house. He wore a black baseball cap on his head that is spotted white with paint. His shoes looked like combat boats that need to be put in the trashcan…yet he had a smile from ear to ear and a happy voice. This was a man you could not tell he wasn't cool. He had a talk and walk of confidence.

He shouted to Mary again: "Put your head up; there is nothing on the ground. Why? Because I picked it all up and smoked it."

Mary could not help but laugh. "Why did you say that?"

"Well, today you look like you lost your best friend so I wanted to make you laugh. I remembered one day I wanted a beer and no one would give me any money. You walked up to me and just out of the blue gave me three dollars and never asked me why or what I needed the money for. I never got the chance to say thank you. So how are you doing today, Miss Lady?"

Now Mary could not tell him the truth—that she wanted a hit of crack and that she had an addiction. All she could do was put her head down in shame as if she was about to cry.

"I'm okay," she responded, but she never looked him in the eye.

Then her inner voice said, *Put your head up, Mary; he already knows your pain.*

Mary asked him, "What is your name?"

"Sam. What's yours?"

"Mary."

With tears running down her face, Mary looked at him and said, "Thank you, Sam, for making me laugh. I sure needed it."

"Well, Mary, come walk with me to the liquor store so I can get my vodka, and let me buy you another beer."

Who would have thought on a day Mary needed a friend, the man she gave one dollar to from time to time would be there when she was at a low point in her addiction.

This is why everyone should be careful how you to treat people, for not only did Sam buy her a beer, he also gave her twenty dollars, a pack of cigarettes, a lighter, and a bag of crack cocaine and never asked her a question or asked her for her body or asked her to come to his house—for Sam was the broker of the neighbor—or, as he would say, he was the consultant of the neighborhood that ran the dungeon.

The things Sam gave her were all the things Mary had just said she wished she had.

Was this bait from the devil? Or was someone or something thing interceding on her behalf?

Little did Mary know her life was about to change. Sam's friendship and the dungeon would become her safe haven.

Wow, what a transformation—if only you could see how it appeared as if she got color back to her skin after Sam gave her medicine. Her tears have now turned into laughter. She is cheerful and uplifted as she begins to walk home after leaving Sam.

Mary gets home and starts dancing around as if she just got her legs. She starts cleaning her house, playing her music. Then she hears a knock on the door.

Okay, is this my high talking or is someone really knocking on my door? Mary says to herself. *Man, every time I'm in my zone somebody is always trying to mess with my high!*

She slowly looks out the window, peeking through the curtain, trying not to be seen.

Damn! It's one of her siblings, crying uncontrollably. Mary puts her drug paraphernalia away, then looks in the mirror to see if she's suitable to be seen and then she opens the door.

"What's wrong? Come in the house. What's wrong?"

Little was Mary ready, for she would get the worst news of her life. She was told her parents were dead.

For Mary, life as she knew it would never be the same. The two people she loved more than life were gone. The two people who understood her and gave her love were now dead.

"Oh my god, oh my god," Mary wailed. "Mama and Daddy are gone!"

Now Mary was left all alone. Yes, she had family, but her mother and father were her life.

Her family never understood Mary and her voices; they never understood the many attempts she had tried to kill herself. Her family never understood the secret pains of her addiction; they never knew that she was a closet addict and had been since she was thirteen years of age.

Now she is in her 30s and Mary is all alone, depressed and full of grief.

With the news of her parents' death, for the first time she did not want to get high despite that she still had drugs to smoke.

All she wanted to do was die to relieve her deep sadness. She started feeling that if she had not been an addict maybe her parents would still be alive. Feeling guilty from the drugs, she began to blame herself.

Mary became felt isolated to her addiction. Now Mama and Daddy were gone; she decided she was going to join her parents so she took an overdose of pills.

Knowing what she had done, Mary got up and walked down the street to Sam's house.

Knock! Knock! Knock!

There was no answer.

Mary knocked again.

Knock! Knock!

Just as she began to leave, the door gradually opened with a creaking sound. This sound reminded Mary of some old spooky movie like *Nightmare on Elm Street, Dawn of the Dead*, or *Psycho*.

All she keeps thinking was *kill! kill! kill!* as if the devil himself was waiting behind the door.

No one answered the door, yet it continued to open. Then a reflection of a person met her eyes at the median of the door, and that person never said a word.

"Hello," Mary began. "May I speak to Sam?"

To her surprise it was Sam at the door. Mary broke into tears and told him her parents were dead, and asked if she could talk to him for a while to get herself together.

This would be the first time Mary would enter the world of the dungeon. This would be the first time Sam had no company in his house.

Who would have thought the closet addict Mary would walk into a world of open drugs and sin? Who would expect Mary the closet addict not to care what other people's opinions would be to see her in such a place? Who would have thought Mary's depression would have total power to make her want to commit suicide? Who would have thought after all the failed attempts as a child on the day her parents died, she would take her life?

But that is what depression does.

On this night, Mary did not care. It was not about her addiction. Maybe she did not want to die alone. Maybe she just needed the comfort of knowing someone cared without a motive. Mary never told Sam she had taken the pills; all she asked of him was if she could rest.

Sam directed her to a secluded part of the dungeon where a couch with several throw pillows on top sat near an old white wall. He took her by her hands and placed a blanket around her as if it was a safety blanket.

But look at this example of mercy in the devil's playground. The example of hope in a dark place of sin was not expected. Sam demonstrated love without a motive to a person who he could have preyed upon in her weakness.

Now let's not forget: Mary felt the need to go into Satan's world to die after taking the pills. Yet never did Sam or Mary think on the night that was meant for evil, God had plans to bring light into a place where people of the church could not go.

For on this night the circumstances in a place of sin, drugs, and death, a friendship of brother and sister emerged, yet someone had to die so someone else could live.

Maybe Sam felt the necessity to help Mary and give her hope because he knew how much she loved her parents. And maybe he understood the impact the death of her parents was going to have in Mary's life and in her addiction.

Sam began to tell Mary everything was going to be okay. He stepped up as if he was her big brother and he assured Mary to rest; he assured her she was safe. All Mary could do was fall asleep, for the overdose of pills was starting to make her sleepy.

Time had passed and visions of light began to cover her eyes then Mary was awakening to the sound of loud talking.

Still not yet fully awake, Mary began to get her thoughts and surrounding in order. For just a short minute she did not know where she was. Then Mary heard Sam arguing with some lady.

Sam's voice was reflecting as if he was an officer in the military: Strong, unfearful, and valiant, he continued to speak and say with his lionhearted voice, "I said LOCK and LOAD!" and the lady proceeded to walk out the door.

As the lady was finally out the door, Sam realized Mary was starting to get up from her sleep.

Mary was shaking as if she was having withdrawals like a person who needed their morning fix of heroin.

She began to take the blankets off that Sam had placed around her shoulders and then she tried to stand up.

"Where am I?" she shouted. "How did I get here?"

Mary had no idea where she was, nor did she have a clue who she was.

Mary began to look around and say in a loud voice, "I am tired of this behavior; this was your last attempt, Mary. Enough is enough!"

Sam looked puzzled. "Are you okay?"

Still confused, Mary began to demonstrate a pugnacious, argumentative, and aggressive behavior as if she was mad at the world.

When Sam started to approach her, Mary responded with a militant voice. "Back the f*** up and keep your hands away from me.!"

Sam was baffled by Mary's behavior, for he never heard her say a curse word before. Sam thought Mary was having some type of hallucination.

Then he began saying, "Hell no! Hold up, wait a minute; it's me, baby girl, Sam. Come back to Earth! Come back!"

All the time Sam was hoping he did not have to call the ambulance or the police to get her out of the dungeon.

He walked over and asked her if she wanted a drink of vodka or a cigarette, he even asked her if she wanted a wake up of crack.

"No!" she responded. "But can I use the bathroom so I can wash my face?"

As Mary was walking toward the bathroom, all she kept saying was "Enough is enough!"

Poor Sam; all he was hoping was he did not have to call the police. *How do you call the police to the dungeon?* he asked himself.

Sam began hearing a different tone in Mary's voice he had never heard before. He started walking toward the bathroom and began to knock on the door.

Knock! Knock! Knock!

"Okay, Mary, who are you talking to?"

The voice continued speaking; repeating the same thing over and over as if it was trying to rationalize an argument.

"All this chick Mary does is keep trying to kill herself over and over! I have had enough! It's my turn, Mary. So goodbye forever."

Sam had no idea what was going on. He knocked on the door again; this time he started shouting, "Get out of my bathroom now!"

"Yeah, okay! I'll be right out."

The door began to open slowly yet she never said a word.

She vacated the bathroom with a new look expressing something was different.

The whole time while she was in the bathroom talking to herself she had created a new look. She had torn the bottom of her shirt in a manner that left the bottom of her stomach exposed. On top of her head she was wearing a matching head wrap from the torn shirt. She had folded the bottom of her jeans like a country girl would do in the country to expose her shoes. Her lips were covered with deep dark red lipstick. She had smeared the same lipstick on top of her eyelids as if it was eye shadow and she used a black eyeliner so dark under her eyes that her natural brown eye color stood out.

When Sam looked at her all he could say was, "This is not the same person." Everything about her—from her voice, her eyes, and her walk—all was different.

Sam was amazed at her transformation of how she looked. "Mary, you had me worried. I thought something was wrong with you. Are you okay?"

Then the silence was broken. She looked at Sam as if she was ready to cut his head off his shoulders.

"Let me get something straight. My name is Pumpkin. That chick Mary is dead. Don't you ever call me Mary again."

Now Sam began to worry and asked, "Who? What did you say your name is?"

"That's right, I said Pumpkin."

Pumpkin began telling Sam that Mary had taken pills to kill herself and that she had come to his house to die. She told Sam in a belligerent voice that Mary was weak and that her time was up. Pumpkin said to Sam, "You won't have any problems with me as long as you respect my name is Pumpkin, not Mary."

Sam was lost for words. Never had he seen a change in personality before. In the dungeon he had witnessed how people reacted once they took a hit of crack cocaine but never had he seen a person who had no drugs or alcohol in their system make such a drastic change.

Little did Sam or Mary know that Mary's failed suicide attempt gave birth to and awakened another personality.

50

Who knows—maybe Mary's alter personality Pumpkin was there all the time. Maybe this alter ego personality had to wait for the right moment such as Mary's failed suicidal attempt and the death of her parents to evolve. Maybe this Pumpkin personality evolved to save Mary, knowing if Mary died she could never exist.

Pumpkin began asking several questions so she could establish the time, the year and her whereabouts.

So who are you? What kind of place is this? What type of relationship do you have with Mary? Why did she feel the need to come here to die?

Sam began to answer Pumpkin's questions, for he did not know how this altered ego was going to react. Sam had been in the military before and he had seen from a combat point of view how trauma can cause amnesia.

The ironic part? Sam welcomed the well-adjusted personality of Pumpkin. He liked the militant, ready-to-fight character Pumpkin displayed after she left the bathroom. Now that Mary the closet addict—the person he had known—was gone, he welcomed the opportunity to mentor Pumpkin because she was green and did not know the drug game.

Sam told Pumpkin he was now officially her family and he reassured her he would not let anything happen to her in his dungeon.

Sam made known to Pumpkin what the dungeon represented and that the dungeon was her new home.

51

He shared with Pumpkin the secrets of his dungeon, how he executed his affairs. He educated her about the creed of the dungeon and all the rules and codes of survival.

He would teach her that she did not have to ask anyone for drugs, beer, cigarettes…not even a cup of water. Sam told Pumpkin, "You are my baby girl and I will take care of you."

His dungeon was the official spot and Sam was the official go to man. During this era of crack, there were several crack houses a person could travel to get drugs. But the dungeon was the spot of very important people. It was not a nickel or dime joint. In order to enter the dungeon you needed a VIP pass.

Sam would tell Pumpkin, "I don't sell drugs but I do sell the VIPs their own fantasy and broken dreams, for if they had money that meant they had no problems paying for the pleasures of crack cocaine."

Sam was the man with the plan. He was the dungeon's overseer.

He knew what a person wanted. He knew where to get what that person wanted and he knew how.

Sam would tell all that willingly entered into the doors of the dungeon, "For the love of money and my consultant fee, the doors of the dungeon are always open."

Yet through all the gloom, sorrow, and wretchedness, he never allowed Pumpkin to see or become involved in the business of the house. She was his baby girl and that meant he instructed all who entered the dungeon hands off and he told everyone to stay away from his baby girl.

People did not like Pumpkin at first. Many could not understand the relationship Sam had with her. Pumpkin could get anything from Sam that other people could not. Everyone who knew Sam was amazed that his relationship with Pumpkin was not intimate.

More and more people began to accept her, for they had never seen Sam so compassionate about a person before nor was Pumpkin used for sexual profit.

Maybe Sam knew somewhere down in Pumpkin's alter soul that Mary was in there. Maybe Sam felt his loyalty was to protect her since Mary trusted to come see him after her parents' death.

Maybe Sam felt his loyalty to Pumpkin was to make sure she would not become lost and turned out, and end up in the wrong hands because of her addiction.

Sam would teach Pumpkin that everyone who entered into his dungeon walked through those doors by their own free will. He would teach Pumpkin this dungeon runs on fat back and cornbread operated by principalities and codes, rules and a creed. Sam would teach Pumpkin that for the love of money, the dungeon doors were always open.

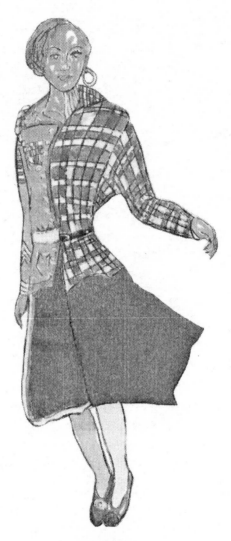

Chapter 3

For the Love of Money

For the love of money is the root of all evil: which while some coveted after, they have erred from the faith, and pierced themselves through many sorrows.
1 Timothy 6 verse 10 { (King James Version}

What can money buy? Is money the key to happiness, prosperity, material possession, or love? For the love of money will a person compromise one's integrity, morals, and principals?

Is money the root of all evil? Or is the love of money the root of all evil?

I wonder: Does money make one become wise? Or for the love of money does one become a fool?

For the love of money, who is in control? I wonder, does money really make the world go round?

Yet we must have it in order to survive. Money is said to have its own character. This lifeless object with its durable qualities has the power to distinguish groups, people, and things from each other. Especially moral and ethical principles that is soon to be replaced by the plastic lifeless debit card.

No matter what anyone wants to believe with money, many fall into sin that leads to addictions. No matter what form of addiction one may have, if it is not recreational, it becomes a habit and from there lack of self-control {addiction} and from there all you have left is misery.

Just ask yourself: Do I have an addiction to drugs, food, alcohol, shopping, cigarettes,

55

prescription drugs, video games, or sex? For the love of money, who wants to admit that?

Greed was one of the seven deadly sins that Satan had released with the S bomb during the crack era. It is a sad fact that money can change people and break up the foundation of families and friends.

Why does money bring greed and envy? Or is the sole purpose of money to bring sadness, pain, and sorrow?

These are the questions the lost souls of addiction face every day. The faces of addiction are not only drug addicts and alcoholics. No, this is far from the truth. Truth is, there are many people that are lost and in bondage to addiction.

For the love of money, for that almighty dollar, it comes to the survival of the fittest. The devil and his demons are not prejudiced about who becomes a slave. It does not matter if you are rich or poor; no one is exempt from falling from the devil's addictions hand.

Google: www. Elite Daily .com for the ten most successful crack heads of all time.

Most addicts try to forget where they were before the life of addiction began. Enslaved by the love of money, many lose motivation and only focus on how to get money to feed their addiction.

For the love of money, it does not matter whether a person has to steal, kill, or destroy. All that becomes important is feeding that addiction. For the addict who needs money for more than necessities, the love of money becomes a personal demon warring against the soul. For the love of money, many have lost hope and faith in a living God all because of sin.

For the love of money, many have lost their minds as well as their lives and for some, money has loved them so much that they are in jail or some kind of institution.

For the love of money, where is Mary? And who is Pumpkin? The fascinating factor of Mary and Pumpkin's dual personality was who truly was the dominant one of the two. It makes you wonder now how Mary got money to buy marijuana at such an early age. It seems as though Pumpkin knew all Mary's business, yet I wonder—was Mary talking to Pumpkin all the time when she was hearing those voices?

Although Pumpkin was different, she learned the value and power of money as well as her self-worth as a person without a true identity, meaning she had no social security number.

Outside of learning who she was, Pumpkin had to try to get some understanding about Mary and see if her addiction, depression, and suicidal behavior affected each other so she would not make the same mistakes.

The ironic part was that Pumpkin got high but her addiction did not affect her in the capacity as did Mary's addiction. Maybe it was because Pumpkin had nothing to hide, whereas Mary the closet addict had to prove to people and her family she worked and did not have an addiction.

Pumpkin accepted she was an addict and for those she came in contact with in the dungeon, she would openly admit, "I am an addict and it is what it is! You don't know me and you don't know my story so let's move on before you judge me."

Just like any addict trapped by addiction, people are going to talk about you. So you better have a game plan or some type of reply. Always keep in mind: misery loves company.

I look at addiction like playing craps or rolling the dice. With the roll of a 7 or 11, you are a winner and you have your addiction under some type of control. But when you roll the dice and get snake eyes, you are a loser and you are at the mercy of your addiction.

Anything and everything goes. Pumpkin knew she had Sam's support, but in the back of her mind she was always thinking, *What if something happens to Sam? How will I survive and feed my addiction?*

One day Pumpkin asked Sam that very question and he in turned began to teach Pumpkin the creed to survival on the street. He would teach her three major principles to remaining alive during the Wild West days of DC.

As long as she followed the creed of the streets, Sam told Pumpkin, she would survive and be all right without him. He would teach Pumpkin by saying, "Don't take any wooden nickel."

One day Sam instructed Pumpkin to create her own personal creed using the words circle, rules, and codes. He told her whatever she wrote down to keep it to herself; he did not want to know what she created.

It took at least a week to complete the assignment, but she did finish and Pumpkin's personal creed went like this:

Rules

ALWAYS be aware and alert
Be aware of who you talk to
Owe no one money
Know nobody
Know nothing
What you do in the dark will come to light
If the person is not beneficial, do not associate
Be careful how you treat people; you never know who you might need
Never trust ANYONE who has an addiction
Be mindful of shadows

Codes

The person you are makes a big difference in the world's addiction
You are an important and valuable person
IT'S BUSINESS, NOT PERSONAL
Know who has your back in the streets of addiction
Never let the right hand know what the left hand holds
The one you think dislikes you is the one you need to watch

Circle

Limit the amount of people you deal with in your addiction circle.

Know who your friends are
Who can you go to if you need something such
as shelter, money, food, or protection?

Pumpkin had to survive and with her militant
attitude and the lesson Sam gave her to creating her
personal creed, she got whatever she wanted within
reason. Pumpkin learned to manipulate people like a
predator that preys on the weak. She would look for
certain persons who could help her without her
being obligated to having sex with them. She would
call them her sugar daddies.

For the bigger picture? It's called survival and
only the strong will survive.

*Google: For the Love of Money by the O'Jays and
let's talk about money and survival at
www.memoirsof2165.com.*

All Pumpkin knew was she did not want to
lose her integrity or let that money or crack become
her god. When I speak of the word integrity I am
reminded of the words from the American journalist
Max Robinson who was the first black broadcast
network news anchor in the United States who died
from AIDS. Max Robinson would leave this Earth
saying, "Never let anybody take your integrity, for
once you lose your integrity, what do you have left?"

For God said, "What do you benefit
if you gain the whole world but lose your own soul?"

After Pumpkin created her personal creed for
survival, she gained a conscience that made her think
differently about life. Maybe that's why Sam
instructed her to create one. Maybe Sam wanted the

60

closet addict Mary to come back. Or maybe Sam wanted more from his baby girl than hanging out at the dungeon. Or maybe it was time for Pumpkin to step out and see what real life was like outside the dungeon walls.

No matter the reasons, Sam knew it was time. He knew she was strong enough to handle life from the streets so he began to engage with Pumpkin concerning all he knew about Mary and her apartment in a place called *The City*.

He told Pumpkin about how Mary's purse had been kept locked away. Both Sam and Pumpkin began going through the purse looking for papers with the address and the keys to the apartment.

Just to think all that time Pumpkin was staying at the dungeon she had a home to go to. Mary had everything in her purse including her ID, her bankcard, social security and birth certificate. She even had pictures of her parents, siblings, and grandmother.

For the first time, Pumpkin almost cried. Sam mapped out her road trip to get to *The City* and he told Pumpkin he could not go; that she had to make this journey by herself. Pumpkin told Sam how grateful she was having him in her life and that she could never repay him for all his kindness and protection.

Sam gave her money and a hug and told her everything was going to be all right. His last instruction to Pumpkin was to be careful and remember, don't take any wooden nickels.

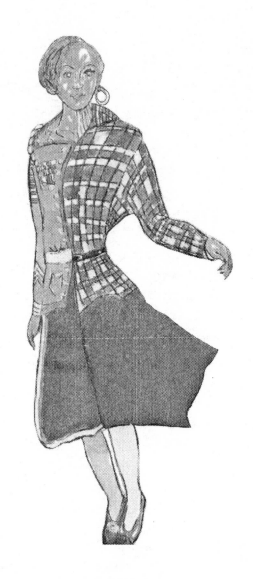

Chapter 4

Oh No, It's Out of Control

Winter was coming and Pumpkin was now in the real world alone. Without life in the dungeon, times were very hard. Being new to the world of drugs alone and without Sam, Pumpkin's life began to turn in another direction and so did her drug use. Although she had sugar daddies who would give her money from time to time, life just did not add up. All that mattered was getting high and trying to escape.

How did I get here? I'm an addict and I am dying and to make matters worse I don't know what I am doing.

Pumpkin was hurting and alone, and the pains of feeding her addiction were calling. Her addiction became her food, her lover, and her best friend.

Pumpkin's appearance was skin and bone, scrawny with a skeletal appearance. She could not have weighed more than ninety-nine pounds soaking wet.

Every time she would look in the mirror, a look of sadness stared back at her—the kind of sadness a person feels when the call of death has taken a loved one.

The mirror revealed the truth that Pumpkin's addiction was out of control. She would ask herself with tears running down her face, *How Lord?* Over and over she would ask, *how did I get here?*

Pumpkin knew her drugs and her addictive behavior became her life. "But why cry?" Pumpkin would say with a sober voice. She would ask herself, "Do I really want to leave the comfort of living this way? I know there is no money, and I know I don't have anyone to love me, but that's okay; my drugs love me."

I know what will make me feel better, she thought as she cried uncontrollably. *I need a hit but I got to find me some money.*

For any addict who understands when there is no money and the addiction is calling, you begin to question your integrity and morals and you begin to wonder if life is worth living.

Pumpkin would ask herself, *Are my tears because I am unable to get high? Or am I crying because I know I am dying?*

Any addict can tell you that in the life of addiction, you have no friends…and everyone has a motive. There was no hope. Pumpkin knew she had to do something to feed the beast, for the devil did not care. He was calling and saying to her, *Feed me and feed me now.*

Addiction is not about your race, color, creed, or sexual preference—for when the devil calls the gambler, the sex, the food, the shopping addict, etc., that call means you better steal, kill, or destroy but you must feed that addiction by any means necessary.

Strung out and unable to function, Pumpkin realized she had to become street smart because she no longer had the safety and comforts of the dungeon. For now she lived in *The City*.

Living in *The City* was different than hanging out in the dungeon. She was all alone in a new environment that was called the devil's playground. *The City* was the pit of hell where the demons would run freely. The people and the spirits are different, and every unclean act against God was permitted. *The City* was a new battlefield of war and Pumpkin did not know any people who lived in her neighborhood.

Before she evolved, Mary had rented an apartment without doing any research of what challenges *The City* offered. The apartment was tiny, a modest looking place that was fairly clean with not too many appliances or furniture. It only had one empty bedroom, with no bed or dresser—just a large framed window.

For a tiny apartment, it had windows all over. There were windows in the kitchen, the hallway, and the bathroom. Each window would allow the sun to peek through the curtains with a rainbow of colors. That seemed to provide the apartment with a warm, sweet, gentle spirit. To put it into words, the apartment had an overwhelming spirit of calmness that assured Pumpkin she was safe as if the spirit of God lived there.

In the living room there was a large beige rosy couch big enough for a person to sleep and use as a bed. Right beside the couch was a little gray radio that had batteries on the floor next to it.

The kitchen and dining room were connected with a refrigerator and there was no table or chairs to have a seat.

The apartment had several closets full of clothes that seemed like they had not been washed. Upon Pumpkin's first visit to Mary's apartment, she went into the bathroom only to learn there was no electricity and the apartment had no heat.

HUM! So this is it? This is my new home. Oh well, it's called survival and only the strong will survive. I just have to make the best out of it.

After Sam had mapped out her journey how to get to *The City,* he instructed her to stay away from the people who lived there. He would advise her of the danger and troubles that lurk in *The City.* He would prepare Pumpkin for a world that was out of control where the devil had full run of the environment. He prepared her, for the people who lived in *The City* were walking zombies.

Sam would tell her *The City* was a city inside of a city, a small neighborhood of run-down industrial buildings and warehouses. He educated Pumpkin of the crimes, prostitution, drugs, and homeless shelters that surrounded the hood. He told her it was one of the poorest wards of DC. He warned her once you entered, it was hard to get out.

He would go on to instruct Pumpkin that *The City* belonged to the devil and he supplied everything a person in addiction would need from sex, drugs, and even death.

Although Pumpkin did not want to live in *The City,* she understood and tried to prepare herself

66

knowing she had nowhere else to go. *The City* was her new home and Pumpkin had to accept she no longer had the protection of Sam or any soldiers or warriors from the dungeon to keep her from harm. She accepted and understood that she could not run over to see Sam every time her addiction was calling.

Pumpkin was getting tired; she knew she had no means to get high so she would stay in the apartment to sleep.

She started sleeping more and crying at the drop of a dime, like a little baby who wants its mommy when it's time to be fed.

One day while sitting on her front porch, Pumpkin saw a friend from the past.

"Hey, Kid, come here! Man, what are you doing in this hood?"

"Hey Pumpkin! What's up with you, baby?"

"Nothing man, I'm just sitting here chilling trying to get a wake up!"

"Oh really?" replied Kid. "You live here in *The City*?"

"Why? You got some drugs, Kid?"

"No girl, I gave that stuff up. I'm on my way to get a bed for the night at the homeless shelter up the street."

"So why did you ask if I live in the hood?"

"Maybe I could invite you to a meeting I attend on Tuesdays and Thursdays."

"What kind of meeting, Kid?"

"It's called NA."

"Oh, you're talking about a drug meeting? Really, Kid, I'm not feeling that right now."

"Okay then, Pumpkin. Maybe one day I can stop by just to check on you."

"Sure, Kid. But before you go can I ask you for a favor? I need a few dollars so I can get me something to eat. I could really use it, man."

Kid slowly reached into his pocket. He pulled out ten dollars and gave it to Pumpkin.

"Wow, thanks man!"

"Now Pumpkin," Kid said, looking into her eyes as he grabbed her hand, "I know what's up. I give you this money because I am your friend. All I am asking from you is for *you* to get something to eat first then do whatever with the rest."

Pumpkin looked into his eyes and said, "Okay, Kid, I will."

Kid, knowing the drug game, never gave her a lecture. He just gave her some street love from a person who understands and knows how it feels to live with an addiction.

Pumpkin held back her tears; she leaned over and thanked him with a kiss on his cheek.

"Hey Kid, what made you stop using drugs?"

Kid turned to look at her solemnly. "There was no more money and my life needed a change.

"Pumpkin, you know there is no loyalty out here in this drug world, so be careful," he continued. "The people you think are your friends are secretly setting you up."

"Hum!" Pumpkin responded. "Yeah, man, you right."

"I'll come back and talk with you soon, so go get yourself together and get you something to eat."

68

Kid walked away waving his hand, as if he knew he would never see Pumpkin again.

Pumpkin watched Kid walk away with a numb feeling of disappointment—she knew once again the beast was calling and the ten dollars was going to be used to feed her addiction, not for food.

Time waits for no one. After seeing Kid, Pumpkin began to stay in the house more. She kept replaying the words Kid said to her about needing a change; those words left a lasting impression on her.

Who knows—maybe the conversation was an awakening for her worthless life. It had been a long time coming. Words can be powerful. Maybe this was the beginning of her change about to come.

Day after day all she wanted to do was sleep and escape from her reality, for sleep became her best friend. Nothing and no one was important. She was depressed and sleep became her first and only priority. Pumpkin was experiencing the kind of sleep where a person feels miserable, down in the dumps, too depressed to get out the bed.

One day while lying on the couch, Pumpkin heard a knock at the window as if the police were knocking on the door.

Knock! Knock!

"Who is it?" she yelled, panic at the edge of her voice.

"It's Bill, come open the door."

Pumpkin answered the door with sleep in her eyes. She had been asleep for several days and never washed her face.

69

Depression has a way to rule your body to one position—maybe two: the bed and bathroom.

"Hay Bill, what up?"

"Girl, I came by to tell you the weather forecaster has predicted an unseasonable, unprecedented cold front is heading toward the East Coast."

"For real, Bill?" Pumpkin answered in a concerned voice.

"Yes!"

Bill was one of Pumpkin's soldiers she met at the dungeon who would stop by from time to time and check on her. He knew Pumpkin did not have any electricity or heat in the apartment. He wanted to warn her that this cold front would be so presidential that the city was making preparation for power failures, broken pipes, and emergency shelters all over the city.

"Pumpkin!" Bill shouted with a strong voice. "Go and wash your face so I can take you to the store to get some candles and something to eat. Go on!"

Pumpkin washed her face and put on some clothes and off to the store they went.

"Hey, Bill, tomorrow is my birthday, are you going to stay for a while?"

"No, I'm going home. I want to be in my house for this snow."

Bill made sure Pumpkin had plenty of candles and matches. He would buy her a sandwich and a large soda to drink to last until the morning. He even gave her twenty dollars.

70

"Happy birthday, Pumpkin. Try to stay in the house tonight and try to stay warm." Out the door Bill went.

Pumpkin was thrilled to get some money. She brought a bag of crack and a beer from the neighborhood bootlegger. Smiling from ear to ear, she had got her legs—a term that addicts use when they are sick from their addiction.

When she got in the house, she began searching for a clean outfit to wear, for she was going to hang at the dungeon for her birthday.

It was the first of the month and everybody was about to get paid in the hood. The drug boys would be selling their dope and the neighborhood convenience stores would be selling their pipes while the tricks and the players were getting ready to get paid.

Pumpkin knew she was about to get some money. Mary had a check coming. Pumpkin was just waiting for it to hit the bank.

While getting ready, Pumpkin heard a loud gust of wind sound hitting against the window. It seemed as if the sound of the wind was blowing through the buildings as if saying, *Stay in the house.*

She looked out the window and there was snow on the ground. Snow was everywhere.

She opened the front door and saw beautiful white crystalline flakes falling from the sky. She looked up and down the street; there were no cars or people moving, just snow everywhere.

Oh no! I got to get out of here and go get my money!

Pumpkin rushed to continue to get dressed, speaking to herself as if someone was in the apartment.

"It's my birthday and it would be crazy to stay in the house tonight alone."

Pumpkin continued talking trying to find logic to convince herself that the weather was not that bad. But the gusty wind was getting stronger and louder; it started sounding like a roaring lion on a hunt.

All of a sudden the candlelight flickered out. She ran to the door to light another candle and with urgency she started checking from closet to closet looking for extra heavy clothing, extra socks, and a hat and gloves to wear to protect her from the snow and the cold weather.

Finally, Pumpkin found all her gear and prepared to head for the door.

All she kept thinking is *It's almost time for Mary's money to hit the bank.*

I got to go now! I refuse to let the snow stop me from hanging out tonight. Nope, not tonight. She walked out her door, saying over and over again, "I got to go! And I got to go now!"

It's funny—when an addict wants to feed their addiction the weather is not a factor. When an addict wants what they want, *nothing* will stop them until they feed that addiction.

Just like Pumpkin the addict, you don't care when that addiction is calling.

Walking had become a struggle, so Pumpkin began to walk in the middle of the street. There were no people or cars moving. No one was walking the empty streets. No one but crazy drug addict Pumpkin trying to get to the ATM machine.

Snow pellets were falling in her face, making it hard to see. It was falling fast, approaching blizzard conditions.

The snow was heavy. It was the kind of snow you could make a snowman, yet the cold temperatures would make it impossible because your hands would freeze before you could get finished. All Pumpkin could think about was getting to the dungeon and getting that first hit.

"I'm going to get high and it's my birthday!" she mumbled to herself in the snow.

This is what having an addiction will do. How can a person in their right mind endure the elements of a snowstorm love themselves? When you have an addiction, you are a slave empowered by the devil.

Pumpkin made it to the main street and was happy to see the neighborhood convenient store was open. She entered the store and wiped off the snow that covered her body and walked over to the ATM machine. She was full of anxiety like a person who gets their first hit.

She reached in her pocket to get her ATM card and went to the machine. Excited, she put the card in, and then she entered the pass code. All she could think about was celebrating—but the ATM machine read insufficient funds.

What!

She tried it again, talking to the machine as if it was a human.

"Come on baby, I need some money!"

Insufficient funds, the machine read again.

No! This cannot be right. Something must be wrong with this machine.

Pumpkin walked to the window where the store attendant was standing.

"Sir excuse me, is this ATM machine working?"

"Yes, miss, the machine is working fine."

"Well, can you help me? I am having a problem getting my money from your machine."

The attendant took Pumpkin's card and swiped it from where he was.

"Miss, please enter your pass code."

Pumpkin hit each number slowly as if she made a mistake at the ATM machine.

"Sorry, miss, there is no money posted on your card; you need to check with your bank."

Hurt and frustrated, Pumpkin began thinking what her next move was. It's almost one o'clock in the morning. "This has never happened before," Pumpkin said, upset and lost. "What am I going to do?"

She left the store and began heading toward the dungeon. The weather was getting worse—the more she walked, the more the snow was beating against her cold face.

Pumpkin's mind started speaking to her, saying, *Girl, you better get to the dungeon fast or you are going to freeze to death.*

Pushing through the heavy snow, Pumpkin arrived at the dungeon.

Knock! Knock!

"Let me in, Sam, it's me Pumpkin."

"Baby girl, what are you doing out here?"

"Man, I need a drink."

Without hesitation, Sam got her some vodka and gave her a cigarette."

The dungeon was empty; only a few soldiers who lived close by were there.

As Pumpkin began taking off her coat, she said, "Sam I need a hit."

"Baby girl, I have a little something. How much money you got?"

Pumpkin was lost for words and with a soft and disappointed voice she looked over to Sam and said, "I don't have nothing." She was nearly in tears. "It's my birthday. My money hasn't hit the bank yet. Somebody give me a phone so I can see if it's been posted so I can go to the ATM machine."

At 1:30 in the morning, Pumpkin called the bank only to learn the money was still not there.

"Baby girl, don't worry I got you, I know you are good for it."

Trying to hold back the tears, Pumpkin said, "Thanks, Sam."

As Pumpkin was in the mist of trying to get high, all she was experiencing was sadness.

Pumpkin's mind was on her money and her own way of celebrating her birthday.

For an addict used to having their own money on the first of the month only to be told insufficient funds, words cannot express the hurt. In her mind, when she left the apartment walking in the snow,

Pumpkin's focus was on spending Mary's money to get her own drugs and come home to get high by herself. Now her plans were broken. She was not in the mood to celebrate. Her depression started setting in and thoughts of frustration took over.

"I'm going home, Sam."

"Why, baby girl? You know you can stay the night."

"I know, I just feel like this is a messed up way to start my birthday off with no money. I don't want to ask anyone for drugs and I don't feel like going through the bull tonight so it will be best for me to go home."

Pumpkin began to get her gear together, looking like a person who had lost their best friend. She proceeded to walk out the door to fight the elements and go home.

As Pumpkin was heading out the door, Sam leaned over and gave her a kiss on her check and said, "Here."

"What's this?" Pumpkin said

He grabbed her hand and gave her ten dollars. "Happy birthday, baby girl." He walked her to the door.

As she began walking in the freezing cold he shouted, "I love you, baby girl, be safe."

Off Pumpkin went. It was so cold that no normal human being should have been out there.

Pumpkin had to endure freezing temperatures to get to *The City*. It must have been ten to fourteen inches of snow that had accumulated. Her hands and feet started becoming numb and her tears were drying like frozen ice.

Pumpkin! Get it together, girl! Her inner voices started encouraging her. *You got to get it together! You must make it home!*

Finally, Pumpkin was close to *The City.* Finally, she made it to her building. Finally, she was in the house.

Tears began to fall from her face. When Pumpkin opened the door a cold breeze hit her harder than the weather outside. She realized she had no heat and no electricity.

What am I going to do?

It was colder in the house than it was outside. Pumpkin ran to find her candles. She opened the kitchen drawer but her hands were wet and frozen, making it impossible to hold the candle, let alone light it.

I need to get out of these wet clothes and find a way to get warm.

She grabbed blankets and clothes, anything she could find in every closet in the house to get warm. She started building a pile of clothes on her couch, placing all blankets on bottom and all kinds of clothing on top. Once everything was in place, she slowly got under the blankets of clothing and began to take off the wet clothes and replaced them with some dry clothing.

All she could do was cry and ask herself, *Why am I living like this? Why Lord did my money not come? Why Lord? Why?*

The cold, hard truth made her wake up to the fact she was an addict and her addiction was her god.

Nothing happens by accident. It just took Mary's money not being posted to face the fact how she really was living.

With no food, electricity, or heat, Pumpkin understood she was at the lowest point in her life. Crying uncontrollably, she shouted, "I'm really an addict!"

It is true—every addict has to travel this road Oh No It's Out of Control alone. Every addict's addiction is different, and every addict's bottom is not the same.

For the first time she realized she had no life and no birth family, and she realized on the day Mary was born she had hit her bottom.

If an addict keeps it real, they can tell you that's what addiction does. It takes you to the bottom, until you want to die with hope to finding peace that seems so far away.

No matter what form of addiction a person has and no matter how good a person you are, addiction has a way to wake you up to see the devastation it has caused to you, your family, and your life.

No one wants to admit they have an addiction. No one wants to admit they are an addict.

Addiction for the addict is a death sentence, and tonight Pumpkin had to admit her way of living had made her life out of control.

There's nothing anyone can say to the person who is lost in addiction that will help them. Yet, until the addict hits their bottom, recovery cannot begin…and until the addict comes to acceptance that their addiction is out of control, the change will never come. No matter what a loved one, a family, or a church will do, *only the suffering addict can make the change.*

Once the addict wakes up and tells themselves, "Okay, I know there is a better way; I remember when life was good; what must I do to be saved and get out before I die?" They are only fooling themselves and everyone who wants them to get HELP!

See, most people with an addiction will tell you that life as an addict was not all bad times. They just got out of control!

When you know it's out of control, there is a sense of hopelessness, sadness, loneliness, and you begin to think of ways to hurt yourself to get rid of the pain. All addicts can tell you when you are in too deep and there seems to be no way out, it's a miserable feeling.

While Pumpkin was lying under the blankets of clothing trying to stay warm, she began to cry. *Enough is enough. I am tired!* Weighed down with tears of hurt and pain, Pumpkin felt like taking a knife to end her life. The cold was starting to affect her mind. With the thoughts of freezing to death, Pumpkin shouted with a loud voice, "I need you, Lord, to answer me before I die in this apartment tonight. HELP ME! HELP ME! Please help me Lord, I am so cold."

Pumpkin realized on Mary's birthday their addiction was sin against God. For the first time, Pumpkin called a Higher Power that Mary knew to call and His name is Jesus the Christ.

For just that moment in the mist of danger and death, Mary evolved and began to pray.

"God! You said *ask* and it shall be given, *seek* and you will find, *knock* and the door will open."

Mary cried out, "Jesus Christ, help me!"

And little did she know He was already waiting for her call. For God will always stand at the door and wait for the person who calls Him. But only Mary could open the door so He could come through.

The Door

I stand at the door and knock anyone that opens the door; I will give him strength and power to overcome that which has enslaved him.

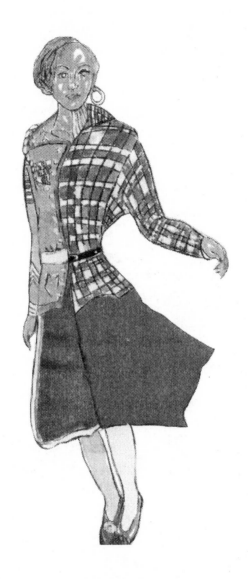

Chapter 5

Please God!

God, it's me, Mary, standing in the need of your help. Please do not pass me by.

Grant me the serenity to accept the things I cannot change, courage to change the things I can and, wisdom to know the difference.

Now that I have been awakened by tears and the shadow of death, I understand what is going on. My heart is still broken and filled with numbness all because my mama and daddy are dead and I just don't want to go on.

Please God, tell me, has my life been a world of fantasy? Have I created a world that only I want to exist? I am trapped within my depression and I am lost in my grief. I am so empty I cannot help but long to be with my mama and I miss the safety of my daddy's arms. Yet, for some reason I am unable to leave this world and free my pain and sorrow.

Why, Lord, did I have to live beyond my last attempt to die? Why, Lord, do I have to keep facing reality?

It is my birthday and it is so cold in this apartment. For the first time I feel death, yet for some reason it seems like someone or some person is counting on me to stay alive.

Could it be I have a purpose bigger than myself? Or is my purpose from my trials and tribulations beyond my own understanding?

Maybe there is a reason why You, God, have interceded so many times so I did not succeed in my attempts of suicide. I know I am weak yet You are strong I am just not ready to face reality.

Please forgive me, God, for being human and not understanding the bigger picture of Your grace and mercy. Please God, can You tell me: Was my awakening the beginning of my renewing process trying to get me prepared for something I have been running from all my life to becoming that person I was always chosen to be?

Then all of a sudden Mary broke into a deep sob. She realized the way she handled her parents' death was the last thing her mother or father would have wanted from her.

God, I know You have always be there for me. I can honestly say You have been the footprint in the sand that has always carried me. Maybe the pain of losing my extended birth family, the drugs, and my feelings of hopelessness are what I am not ready to bear.

Please God, forgive me.

Just as Mary finished her prayer with God, Pumpkin woke up and it was morning.

Removing her shelter of blankets and clothing, Pumpkin saw a beautiful ray of light peeking through the curtains. From every window there was a ray of colors that radiated warmth that created heat through the apartment.

Little by little she would remove each layer of clothing until she reached the warmth of the light that radiated from the sun rays, which provided her with a sense of hope from an unexplainable source of heat as if someone had turned the heat on in the apartment.

Pumpkin got up with a smile on her face, for she knew she had made it through the bitter, arctic night. Her smile and the sun's rays were confirmation she was still alive.

Pumpkin walked into the bathroom and looked out the window to see the most amazing sight: The sun was shining bright and gleaming on the snow; it seemed like a ball bouncing up and down from the reflections of light. The reflection seemed as if the snow was inviting you to come outside and play and enjoy its unique beauty.

Wow! I made it through the night, Pumpkin thought to herself. Never once did she realize what occurred while she was sleeping.

She left the bathroom and walked into the kitchen to be welcomed by the most amazing sight. On top of the refrigerator was a book illuminated by a ray of light shining through the window, beckoning her as if she was being directed to pick it up.

Pumpkin never questioned the mystery of the invitation; she just went to the refrigerator and picked up the book.

As would be appropriate and not a coincidence, it was the Bible and the words that were written for Pumpkin to read on such a day as Mary's birthday.

She opened the Bible and the first scripture she came to was Psalms 62, which was marked and circled with red ink that started from verse 5.

She began to read the Bible out loud as if it were God's voice speaking to her:

My soul waits thou upon God: for my expectation is from him.
He only is my rock and my salvation: he is my defense; I shall not be moved.
In God is my salvation, and my refuge, is in God. Trust in him at all times; ye people, pour out your heart before him: God is a refuge for us. Se-lah

"Thank You, God, for allowing me to wake up this morning, and thank You, God, for allowing me to live through the night. Thank You for giving me another chance. Please search my heart and

85

direct me in the way I should go," Pumpkin murmured.

Then to Pumpkin's surprise she began to shout halleluiah and repeatedly continued to thank God, for on this new day God was preparing Pumpkin to meet Mary's family as someone who Mary's family did not know existed.

Pumpkin proceeded to the bathroom to get herself together. While washing her face she looked in the mirror and began to say to herself, *How can I go to Mary's family looking like this?* The mirror revealed her eyes puffed up from crying and her face sunk in from the abuse of her addiction and depression. For the first time since she evolved, Pumpkin was ready to face reality even though she did not like the way she looked in the mirror.

She remembered the words from the Serenity Prayer and asked God for courage, and out the door she went. While heading down the street walking in the snow, all she kept thinking was *I am alive, I made it through the night.* She was trying to convince herself she was doing the right thing in facing the unknown.

Pumpkin was getting closer to Mary's parents' house and her fear began to kick in. She questioned herself: *This is a bad idea,* she thought. *I will do it some other time; I'm going home.*

But she was too close to turn back now; Pumpkin was right across the street. She could hear laughter and smell bacon and all types of food aroma that made her stomach growl. Pumpkin knew she was hungry so she said, "I am going to knock on the door."

Just as she knocked on the door, the door swung open and the people in the house stopped laughing and began to say, "Mary, it is you! Happy birthday!"

Then all of a sudden everyone started rushing to the door and kissing her and giving her hugs and telling her how much they missed her.

"Wow!" was all Pumpkin could say. The love and the acts of kindness she felt were overwhelming, for this was something new and what she had been missing since she evolved.

She looked around to find a seat and proceeded to take off her coat. Someone from the family said, "Mary, why do your eyes look like that? What have you been doing? Have you been up all night getting high?"

Pumpkin did not say a word. Then someone asked her, "Have you lost weight? You look like skin and bones." Again Pumpkin did not say a word.

Holding back her sharp tongue, Pumpkin just took their questions and said to herself, *This is the devil trying to steal my happy moment of joy.*

Then someone else asked her, "What's wrong with you, Mary? Where have you been?"

Not knowing how to answer all the questions, Pumpkin maintained her composure, looked everyone in the eye, and began to say, "Hello everyone, my name is Pumpkin."

You could hear a pin drop on the floor while all the laughter had stopped.

The family was shock and began to laugh at her, saying, "You are crazy. Who the hell is Pumpkin?"

If only you could have been a fly on the wall to see the disappointment, hurt, and pain revealed on Pumpkin's face. Yet she did not say one word. The family told her whatever type of drugs she was using made her lose her mind and that it was time for her to leave. To make matters worse, they told Pumpkin they did not want to know her. However, they did tell her when Mary came back to let Mary know she would always have her family.

Sad and lost for words, Pumpkin left the house crying, hurt, and hungry. *I need a hit that will take this pain away*, she thought to herself. Yet keeping it real that's not what Pumpkin wanted; all she really wanted and needed was understanding and love.

She wanted the love, the hugs, and the kisses she received when she walked through Mary's parents' house. She wanted the emotional love she received just for that short moment—something she had been yearning and missing. Something drugs have not been able to give her.

Let's talk…. No matter how much drugs a person uses to escape from hurt and pain, it seems you can never get high enough to forget. There is no addiction or sex or money that can replace love. Maybe it can give you that temporary feeling of comfort; however, it cannot give you LOVE!

While walking and heading toward *The City,* Pumpkin began to experience emotions that were locked inside of her. She began to question herself and her self worth after Mary's family rejection. While walking down the street, a cold wind started pushing her closer to home as if it was the devil calling and welcoming her back to the lost city and the lost people, as if this was the only life she deserved.

Rejection is the worst thing to experience when someone is hurting and searching for love. Rejection is what the pimp or predator will use on the weak person and give those fake dreams and fake feelings of love. Rejection is one of the root keys to addiction and one of the main reasons why so many people use drugs and alcohol to escape the emotions associated with rejection, hurt, and pain.

Pumpkin would learn on the day Mary was born she had no one to love her, for she really did not exist. It was easy for her to be militant and hard. It was easy for her to use drugs as her defense to having no emotions. Yet Pumpkin, just like most addicts, realized there comes a time in an addict's addiction when you must face life on life's terms.

The grips of addiction can take an addict through many emotions, but today after her rejection Pumpkin did not want to numb her emotions. She wanted to remember the amazing love she felt when she first woke up and how God told her to trust in Him, for it was His love why she survived the bitter cold night.

She knew once she made it back to *The City*, Satan and his demons would give her a free high to forget Mary's family and a free high to trap her to forgetting how God brought her through.

She knew the devil was not going to let her go without a fight.

For any addict wanting to make a change in their life from addiction, it will be difficult. I don't care how many times you convince yourself; today is the day I will no longer be a slave to drugs, or alcohol, or gambling, or porn/sex or eating, or shopping, or prescription drugs...it will not happen in a day and anyone that tells you something different is liar and the truth is not in them.

One should be careful and learn the motive, the source, the reasoning or theory of a person that states it is easy to quit. There is no easy way to leave the life of addiction; it is a process.

Pumpkin made it to the apartment safely and was grateful. She had no clue what was going to happen next. Pumpkin took off her clothing and began to cry. *Lord, I have no one but You to call. Please God, I don't want to use drugs today. I don't want to feel the pains of rejection anyone. I am all alone and I am hurting. Yet I don't want to die, for the night is coming soon and the cold will return in this apartment. Help me, God. Please help me!* With tears running like a river down her face she prayed to God.

Then all of a sudden someone began to knock at her window.

Knock! Knock! Knock!

Pumpkin wiped the tears that were falling from her face and wiped her running nose. *Who could this be knocking on the window?* Pumpkin asked as if she was afraid to answer the door. Then she began to laugh: *Okay, God! Is that you knocking on the window?*

You should have seen the smile on her face. She was smiling as if the answers to her prayers were knocking on the window right after asking God for help.

The knocks got louder and they seemed to get harder, making Pumpkin upset.

She yelled out, "Who is it!? Why are you knocking on my window like that?"

"It is Teacher."

"Who is Teacher and what do you want?"

Now let's not forget Pumpkin has not been high all day. Who knows—Teacher could be the man sent from the devil to get her high.

Addiction has a way to trap you, however when you are truly asking for help never be afraid to open the door—it could be the help you are praying for. So Pumpkin went and opened the door.

"How are you doing, Miss Lady?"

"I am doing fine," Pumpkin responded. "Please forgive me, sir, where do I know you from?"

Teacher laughed and asked Mary, "Why are you acting like you do not know who I am?"

"Really, sir, I don't have a clue." Little did Pumpkin understand, Teacher was a friend of Mary's. It had been fifteen years since they last seen each other. Teacher would begin to tell Pumpkin God told him to find her and help show her the way of escape.

Teacher had just come home from a place where addicts could go and get help for their addictive disorders called rehab.

Teacher would share with Pumpkin information concerning how God wanted her to get into a drug treatment program. All Pumpkin could do was cry; she could not believe the God of mercy could love her and send help just like that. For Teacher to find Pumpkin right after she had prayed for help was nothing but God's work.

Teacher told her she had nothing to be ashamed of, that all have sinned and come short of the glory of God. But it was time for Mary to face her demons and secret pains.

Teacher would share and comfort Pumpkin that God heard her prayers and he wanted her to know it was time for Mary to come back. Mary had turned away from God and her sins were bringing judgments. Teacher began to stress to Pumpkin the importance of the message God told him to deliver and why she must leave with him and go to a place called Addiction Prevention Recovery Administration, APRA, to get help because her life depended on it.

Teacher began to talk of his faith by telling Pumpkin that faith is the substance of things hoped for and the evidence of things not seen. He would give her understanding and hope that God opens doors in spite of what anyone has done.

Teacher would say rehab was the best thing that happened to him and how his mind is clear to see things differently. Then he looked at her and he asked Pumpkin, "Are you ready to go?" Never once did he call her Mary. It was as if Teacher was meeting Pumpkin where and who she was in her life.

In between the tears Pumpkin answered him and said, "Yes, I am ready to go to rehab!"

Pumpkin made sure everything was in order and locked the apartment door. All she had with her was Mary's identification.

On the day Mary was born, through the rejection and demonic environment of *The City*, God truly showed Pumpkin He was alive.

Teacher would take Pumpkin by the hand to make sure she got in rehab that day. He waited with her during the registration time and he waited until she got on the bus to leave.

With tears in her eyes as she was getting on the bus, Pumpkin leaned over to thank Teacher and tell him how grateful she was that she did not have to sleep another night in *The City* or stay in that cold apartment with no utilities. She would thank him for waiting with her and saving her life.

As the white bus left the parking lot, Pumpkin would cry uncontrollably with tears of joy and a heart full of peace.

Before leaving, Teacher told Pumpkin that she was going to a detox rehab center that was really a psychiatric ward. He said to her, "Do not be afraid. Just get ready and prepare yourself to face the truth what Mary was running from and to learn who Pumpkin really is."

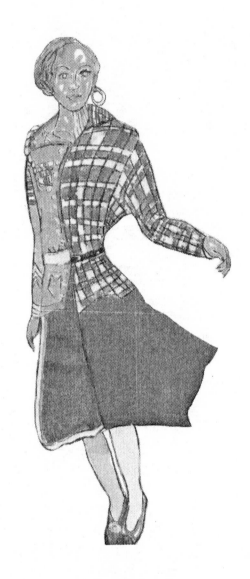

Chapter 6

Psych Ward here I Come

Psych Ward Here I Come would be the beginning for Pumpkin to get the right help for her addiction through a variety of treatments from psychiatric inpatients, outpatient behavioral treatment, drug rehab programs, group counseling, and professional therapy.

Psych Ward Here I Come is for the person who is ready to surrender the old way of living with the understanding that recovery from addiction and mental health issues they can be professionally addressed.

When Pumpkin arrived at the detox psych ward, she did not know what to expect. Teacher tried to educate and encourage Pumpkin not to be afraid and to welcome the help.

Although she was somewhat afraid of the unknown, Pumpkin was relived to be there, for all Pumpkin knew she did not want to die or go to jail or visit the grave early because she had seen firsthand living in *The City* those are the effects of addiction. For the first time, Pumpkin's mind and body were in for a rude awaking. She made it through a whole day clean and sober.

The hospital staff was helpful and friendly once she arrived to the detox by showing her to her room. Once she got settled in, a loud announcement came through the speakers saying group time was to commence. New to her surroundings, Pumpkin would ask herself, *What is group time? I hope I do not have to attend; I just got here.* All she wanted to do was go to sleep. Her mind and body were so tried.

Just as she was about to lie down, someone knocked on the door and then the door quickly opened. It was the hospital nurse who would inform her she had to attend the group session.

The nurse explained to Pumpkin the purpose why the hospital engaged in group sessions and why she must attend the first group.

"But I am so tired," Pumpkin said.

The nurse continued to encourage Pumpkin. Although she was tired, the group session would give her a chance to see other people and learn she was not alone.

Tried, afraid, and fearing the unknown, Pumpkin decided to attend. To her surprise the room was full of people from all age groups and racial backgrounds. It was like a town meeting.

The group leader began the session with the rules of the group and educated the group on what to expect while they were in the detox ward.

The leader had no cut cards about the truth and told the group what the body was about to encounter emotionally and physically. Right from the beginning, the leader expressed, "If you want help while you are here, the hospital will do everything to help any patients just as long as the patients would be true to thyself and accept a treatment plan."

"Wow, all this tonight?" Pumpkin asked the leader.

With all eyes on Pumpkin, the leader answered her with a soft voice, "Did your addiction happen in a day?"

Embarrassed by the question, Pumpkin answered no.

The leader asked Pumpkin if she would like to share her story with the group. With her head held down, she replied, "No, I am not ready."

After the group session was over, embarrassed by all the eyes on her, Pumpkin walked to her assigned room with her head held down. Upon entering into the room, Pumpkin noticed a short, brown haired woman. Not being in the mood to be friendly, Pumpkin walked around the woman and went to her bed, when she heard another announcement over the speaker.

ATTENTION! ATTENTION! Dinner is about to be served.

"Wow, how does one get sleep around here?" Pumpkin mumbled.

Her roommate began to laugh and asked Pumpkin, "What, are you not hungry?"

Pumpkin answered the woman, "I am so tired I just want to sleep."

"Then go to sleep," the woman said. "By the way, my name is Nicki; you go ahead and get some rest. I'll tell the staff you are not ready to eat." She turned off the light and left the room.

Just as Nicki exited, Pumpkin started to feel sick. Maybe it was the fact she had no drugs or alcohol in her system and her body was feeling it.

Pumpkin's body was starting to remove harmful toxins. She was in the beginning stages of withdrawal with symptoms of anxiety, agitation, sweat, nausea, tremors, paranoia, and vomiting. Who knows, maybe walking in the snow the night before got the best of her body.

Just at the moment Pumpkin was about to vomit, Nicki walked in the room and observed Pumpkin was sick.

"Are you alright?" Nicki asked.

Pumpkin could not say a word. Nicki walked her to the bathroom and called for help.

Pumpkin began to cry and said, "Thank you, Nicki, for helping me."

All of a sudden Pumpkin started to remember her creed: *Be careful how you treat people; you never know who you might need.*

All during the night Nicki would help Pumpkin and she would never leave her side.

The next day Pumpkin was awakened by the most amazing sound of singing birds. Pumpkin was so glad to have made it through the night.

Then she heard Nicki say, "Good morning, Pumpkin, how are you feeling?"

"Good morning Nicki. It's a beautiful day to be alive."

"Well Pumpkin, it is time to go eat breakfast and attend a morning meeting. So come on and get yourself ready."

Pumpkin just wasn't in the mood and she was still feeling sick, so she asked one of the staff nurse at the desk if she could miss the group session.

"No, this is a mandatory meeting," the nurse kindly stated, then told her that since Pumpkin was a patient, going to the group session was a part of her treatment.

Pumpkin returned to her room to shower and get dressed.

After breakfast, both Nicki and Pumpkin went to the room before the mandatory morning meeting. Nicki asked again, "How you are feeling? Girl, you scared me last night, you really was sick huh?"

"Yes I was," Pumpkin wailed, then began to cry.

"Why are you crying?"

Pumpkin wiped her tears and began to tell her it was a long story as she wiped the tears falling from her face. Pumpkin asked Nicki how long had she been in detox.

"I have been here for a week and tomorrow I am going home." Nicki told Pumpkin they could talk more once the morning meeting was over and asked Pumpkin, "Are you ready to go? I will walk with you so you don't have to feel alone."

"Thanks Nicki, I am ready."

"Good morning, everyone. My name is Nurse *Get Yourself Together.*"

All you could hear was laughter.

"What kind of name is that?" Pumpkin asked. "Who might you be?"

Again Pumpkin put her foot in her mouth. "My name is Pumpkin."

The nurse replied, "Well, Pumpkin, let's begin the meeting with information about the detox center, why you are here, and what happens to the body. Then if anyone has questions or wants to share, the meeting will be open for all discussion."

Nurse *Get Yourself Together* began the meeting saying, "See, Pumpkin, you must be open to the tools of learning and listening, understanding the purpose of your individual treatment plan, as well as the group sessions that will educate you here at the detox psych ward.

"You are free to walk out anytime you choose; however, you must remember for anyone that has not been through detoxification, your body will go through many emotional and physical changes. The purpose to start the recovery process at the detox psych ward is so the hospital can monitor the patients' withdrawal symptoms and keep a watch for any behavioral changes such as suicidal ideations and how the detoxification will affect your body."

Pumpkin had to keep in mind that Mary started using drugs at an early age, which added years of abuse to the body, mind, and spirit. Just two days clean, her body was already releasing toxins that added to her feeling sick.

The detox psych ward was a place with psychiatrists and health professionals who not only dealt with recovery from addiction, but they were also trained to identify mental disorders such as:

Schizophrenia disorders
Bipolar disorders
Anxiety disorders
Childhood disorders
Cognitive disorders
Dissociative disorders
Eating disorders
Impulse control disorders
Mood disorders
Personality disorders
Sexual disorders
Sleep disorders

For most addicts, the fight to stay clean and sober will come with a price, but be encouraged—addiction is change behavior. It is a process to living.

Nurse *Get Yourself Together* continued to say it is recovery turned to the right with a different insight to life. "While you are here at the detox center, take advantage of the group sessions that will give each person a chance to listen as well as participate. There is a wealth of information in this room. People can talk about their medication as well as places where you could go get help with problems, and you can network here, too. If you don't remember anything else while you are here, just remember you are not alone. There is hope. Are there any questions or would someone like to share?"

Everyone glanced around at each other but no one answered.

"Alright then, the meeting is over. Have a great day."

"Wow, what a great morning meeting," Pumpkin said.

"That's how all the meeting are here," Nicki said, grinning at her.

"Do you like attending group?"

Nicki explained to Pumpkin why the group sessions were important and how the staff really educated and encouraged the patients there. "Girl, I have received information where to find programs, places for food, clothing, and shelter once I leave. All the staff asks is for the patients here to give recovery a chance." Nicki walked over, sat on Pumpkin's bed, and said, "You will find people with addiction and mental health disorders are more alike than different. I have learned if I give truthful answers to understanding why my life is unmanageable then my process of recovery can and has begun. Girl, you are going to be amazed how many people you are going to meet who are suffering from of all forms of addiction. Many people here have suffered from trauma, neglect, physical, and mental and emotional abuse. They've just never dealt with it; they have only self-medicated through drugs and alcohol."

Nicki would encourage Pumpkin to always remember the group session is the way any addict can reach one and teach one how to get your life back. Nicki took Pumpkin by the hand and said, "I

102

am so grateful for the detox psych ward and I welcome going to the thirty-day drug rehab program. See, today I desire to live and not die anymore from my life as an addict trapped by my addiction."

As Nicki finished talking, the announcement came over the speakers. It was lunchtime.

Listening to Nicki gave Pumpkin much to think about. Asking Pumpkin to change from her comfort zone of drugs was new, only she could make that choice and only she had to want it. That goes for any addict—no one can convince you. The person with addiction and mental health {co-occurring disorders} must want it first.

Society, family, and friends must learn and accept the truth that the more you ask the addict to enter into treatment and seek help, the more the addict will run away to escape into their addiction.

I am here to tell you that you can talk until your face turns blue, just always remember for any addict trapped by depression, rejection, failure, and despair, their addiction will always be their comfort and their addiction will always come first.

The only reason Pumpkin was at the detox center was because God was knocking on the door, Mary's first of the month check wasn't posted, and the snowstorm knocked her down.

While eating lunch, Pumpkin sat at a table near the window. She looked at the snow that was starting to disappear. A smile of joy came upon her face, for she realized how grateful she was for Nicki's insight and help. She would say to herself, *Maybe I should be quiet and listen more.*

After lunch, Pumpkin went to her room to take a nap. She felt a peaceful spirit entering into the room and began to fall into a deep sleep.

After her nap, she looked and felt better than ever before. She was safe and warm and she was alive.

"Wow! You got some rest," Nicki acknowledged with a cheerful voice.

"Yes, I did," Pumpkin replied, "and I am hungry. Is there anywhere I could get a clean hospital scrub to wear to dinner, Nicki?

"Sure! I'll go get one from the nurse; I'll be right back."

Once Pumpkin felt fresh and happy, the two ladies left the room and went to eat dinner.

Nicki and Pumpkin sat together with two other patients.

"Hello everyone," one of the ladies at the table said to Nicki. "Did you hear that at tonight's meeting we are going to have a guest speaker?"

"Who?" Nicki asked.

"I am not sure, but they say she is a powerful motivational speaker."

After dinner all the patients gathered together to meet the guest speaker, a former addict who came to visit and share her story of recovery. She had a powerful testimony on how her life had changed and the steps she was doing to stay clean and sober. She never talked about her past; she just encouraged everyone listening about her faith, love of self, and her life from people, places, and situations.

She opened the floor to questions and asked if anyone wanted to share. No one wanted to talk, but then suddenly Pumpkin raised her hand to speak.

"Hello," she began in a deep, saddened voice. "My name is Pumpkin and I am an addict. I do not know who I am or how I got to this point in my life, all I know is I want to live so I'm here at the detox psych ward asking for and seeking help. On the first of the month, I tried to celebrate this person who is locked inside of me named Mary's birthday. We share the same body yet we are so different."

With tears running down her face, Pumpkin stood and said, "As of today, I would like to be called Mary/Pumpkin and if it is alright with the group, I would like to share a story."

The guest speaker held her arms out and hugged Pumpkin so she would not be afraid.

As she began to speak, her voice cracked as if she was holding back the truth. Then, with a soft tone, she told the group about a re-occurring dream she had of living in a dark hole that had no light and how she would hear voices trying to point her to the way out, and how many times she would run to the voice but could never get out of the dark hole.

She told the group once she could see the light she would run away because of fear. Then she began to cry as if she was freeing her soul and told the group, "My name is Mary and I have been lost for so long. I would run and run and hide so no one could find me. I now understand why Pumpkin evolved. She came to save me from death.

105

"I saw the light and I was not ready to deal with the trauma in my life so Pumpkin walked toward the light and took over all to save me so I could live. I know it sounds crazy; maybe that's why I'm here at this psych ward."

With tears running down her face she continued: "My name is Mary/Pumpkin and I forgot how to live and who I was. I have been gone for so long."

While wiping the tears, Mary said, "Thanks; I feel so much better."

For the first time, Mary the closet addict was ready to accept the wrong in her life and was willing to do whatever it would take to be the person her parents raised her to be. She was now ready to deal with her addiction and understand Pumpkin along with accepting she had hit her bottom.

After the group session, the guest speaker approached Mary/Pumpkin and told her how she enjoyed her testimony and asked her if they could have a private meeting in the next room. Apprehensive Mary/Pumpkin went.

The guest speaker kindly said to Mary/Pumpkin, "Now that you have accepted who you are, I would like to share something with you, so please keep an open mind to the things I am about to say.

"In order to stay clean and sober, you must have balance in your life. You must learn to depend on a higher power to guide you through this new way of living. You must learn to trust God."

For God gave us a spirit not to fear, but of power and love and self-control.
2 Timothy 1:7

"See, Mary, once you surrender your life to God, He can and will use you for greater work, for all you have been through is so you can share your testimony of the power of God. You will be able to tell someone how God never forgot you."

The guest speaker took Mary/Pumpkin by the hand and shared, "For the battle is not yours; it is the Lord's. You must understand from this day forward the enemy cannot do anything to you unless he gets God's permission.

"While you are here at the detox psych ward, learn as much as you can about your co-occurring disorder. Learn the necessary tools to live life clean and sober. You must understand recovery is a process; you will not always win but never give up.

"Never beat yourself up when you relapse because you will relapse. *It is a part of recovery.* Call on your higher power and He will give you all you need.

"Last thing to remember, Mary/Pumpkin: You cannot run away from yourself or your problems. Seek one-on-one therapy and learn more about who you are. Yes, today you are Mary/Pumpkin, but do you really know who you are?"

The guest speaker would share with her that one-on-one therapy would help unlock the mind so an individual can deal with the demons of the past and allow God to set them free. "Today you are

Mary/Pumpkin, but in order to live a life clean and sober, Pumpkin has to go.

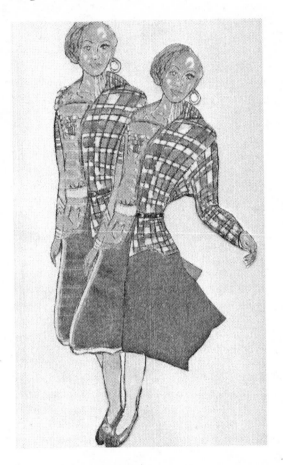

"In order to win in your addiction, you must decide between yourself and face the demons of the past to get the answers to the question who is Mary? And who is Pumpkin? It will be hard to face, but if you want to live, you must understand you no longer will be able to use your past addictions as a familiar pattern to deal with life's disappointments. It can only be one winner—Mary or Pumpkin."

Mary/Pumpkin thanked the guest speaker and went to her room where Nicki was packing her clothes so she could go to the drug rehab center the next day.

"So your name is Mary/Pumpkin? How are you doing? Girl, you said some powerful words tonight and I would like to thank you. Your story touched my heart. Listening to you has given me the push I need."

Mary/Pumpkin and Nicki gave each other a hug, said a prayer, and went to sleep.

The next day Mary/Pumpkin woke up to find Nicki was gone. On the table was a letter and a flower plant that Nicki wanted her to have. The note read: *God will never put more on you than you can bare; never stop believing in yourself, maybe one day we will meet again. Until then, stay focused. Your friend, Nicki.*

After Mary/Pumpkin came from breakfast, she was asked to come to see the psychiatrist to discuss her treatment plan. Mary/Pumpkin's treatment plan would include:
Stress management
Medications management
Understanding what her triggers are
Relapse prevention
Anger management
Co-occurring trauma education

The psychiatrist at the hospital instructed Mary/Pumpkin that her treatment plan would begin here at the detox psych ward but she must continue to seek help in a thirty-day drug program and after that she would be advised to seek an outpatient day program.

The psychiatrist would educate her on what co-occurring disorders are and how these disorders were readily treatable by using adjunctive methods, medications, and psychotherapy.

The psychiatrist told her that in general, the sooner a problem is identified and addressed, the better the chance of recovery. Mary/Pumpkin was instructed that she would have to accept what her beginning drug abuse was, then gain understanding of her past thinking and behavior so she could get to the truth that directly led her to having mood swings, anxiety, and depression.

She would also have to find what was needed to work on the change so she could identify and properly treat each condition.

Mary/Pumpkin learned that if she could not identify stress and properly treat each condition, it would interfere with and complicate her overall efforts to recover.

The psychiatrist concluded that when she was physically stable and ready to address other concerns, she would need to develop a conflict resolution that would help her. "You need to understand what is stress management and must learn coping strategies so you can manage and learn how to address positive feelings of being in control of your life," she said.

While at the detox psych ward, Mary/Pumpkin would learn the beginning stages of promoting her general well-being. Mary/Pumpkin understood that she needed to learn not to bottle her feelings up. If something or someone was bothering her, she had to face and learn how to communicate her concerns by figuring out what she could do to deal with unhealthy stress as well as the normal everyday stress of family jobs or living life on life's terms. Mary/Pumpkin's treatment plan also included her keeping a daily journal to learn how to adjust her attitude and manage her stress.

By writing in her journal, she would learn how to identify self-defeating thoughts. She would learn what effects would have on her emotional and physical well-being.

The detox psych ward would educate her that each time she would think a negative thought about herself that her body would react to that situation.

Mary/Pumpkin had to learn that if she could see good things about herself, she would feel better about herself. She had to teach herself to get in a habit of eliminating negative words and not allow herself to dwell on the bad parts of the past.

Mary/Pumpkin's treatment plan would also include relapse triggers that involved people, places, things, and situations.

Since Mary and Pumpkin used drugs and alcohol to soothe her feelings, Mary/Pumpkin would have to understand, identify, and learn her limitations. She would have to gain understanding that breaking a drug or alcohol habit is not easy and is going to have ups and downs. She had to accept that Relapse Triggers happen to people if they do not remove the bitterness or regret of the past. She had to accept if she did not remove them she would remain stuck in addiction.

The psychiatrist also told Mary/Pumpkin that as long as she did not face the past or as long as she was feeling too ashamed to seek professional help, she was setting herself up for failure. Pumpkin was instructed to seek a sponsor and support group.

Each day Mary/Pumpkin gained more insight to recovery. It was as if she was a newborn baby giving a chance to walk or that big girl ready to ride her bike without training wheels.

On one of her meetings with the psychiatrist, Mary/Pumpkin was asked what faith was she and did she believe she deserved to live a new way of life? She never gave any responses, but instead she just listened to what the doctor had to say.

Mary/Pumpkin would have to learn that she could not be mad at herself or anyone else. She had to forgive family, friends, and the individuals who played a part in her addiction.

Just as the psychiatrist talked about relapse triggers, Mary/Pumpkin interrupted and said, "I guess I could continue to let the people who hurt, used, and abused me be my reason to continue to get high once I leave the detox psych ward, huh?"

She lowered her head and began to cry. "What must I do to win in recovery; how do I not be afraid to want to run or escape? To me, not running from reality it all sounds so new. I know I must learn to identify my relapse triggers so I can move from the past and begin by starting fresh. I'm tired now and I am willing to take this walk of faith."

The nurse and psychiatrist staff was so proud to hear Mary/Pumpkin say that they would comfort her by educating her more, saying, "As you walk this road of recovery, learn to identify early the underlying causes and warning signs of past trauma, stress, and anxiety that would and could create addiction craving.

"If you let personal issues such as fearing going home become your crutch, you are far more likely to return to your bad habits. Know this, Mary/Pumpkin: Your treatment plan is a plan that will take time. Do not get overwhelmed; we are here to assist you with the tools you will need, and once you go to the thirty-day program, you will learn more and have clean time from your addiction. You are doing well. Just don't give up!

The next day, Mary/Pumpkin met with the treatment nurse staff to talk about her medication for her co-occurring disorder. Now Mary/Pumpkin was aware that she suffered from an undiagnosed condition of depression, which was one of the causes of her suicidal behaviors along with the hearing of voices that she would talk to.

The importance of medication management in the psych ward is to identify and help manage

113

Schizophrenia disorders
Schizoaffective disorders
Bipolar disorders
Anxiety disorders
Childhood disorders
Cognitive disorders
Dissociative disorders
Eating disorders
Impulse control disorders
Mood disorders
Personality disorders
Sexual disorders
Sleep disorders

Mary/Pumpkin learned to never stop using her medications that were prescribed unless advised by her professional doctor, even if she was feeling better. The psychiatrist and nursing staff would also educate her that some prescriptions are there to help you get past the dangerous side effects of withdrawal. She was instructed to always let her doctor know of all bodily changes.

The last part of her treatment plan was anger management. The psychiatrist and nursing staff asked her if she knew what the elements of anger were in her addiction, and when she said no, they proceeded to educate Mary/Pumpkin. The psychiatrist and nursing staff would explain that anger is often a cover-up for other feelings and a mask to cover up unaddressed past issues, or in other cases, anger was used as an excuse to manipulate others.

The psychiatrist and nursing staff told Mary/Pumpkin in order for her to move forward she had to get in touch with herself and learn how to express her anger in appropriate ways.

The psychiatrist and nursing staff handed her another journal and pencil and told her to write in her journal every day what she was feeling.

The psychiatrist and nursing staff educated her to pay attention to the way anger makes her body feel and pay attention to the negative thought patterns. She was also educated to be prepared to understand the insensitive actions of others by learning how to interpret and think about the situations and causes to make you become frustrated and angry that will lead you to wanting to get high or go back to your addictive behavior.

In a short time, Mary/Pumpkin realized that her addictions, judgment, and actions with both personalities from Mary and Pumpkin were a major force to her anger. She understood her negative anger impacted the way people saw them both.

Boy was Nicki right, Mary/Pumpkin would say to herself while she was writing in her journal.

Here at the detox psych ward, Mary/Pumpkin would learn in the group sessions not to admit you are an addict or have a mental illness to make someone feel better. Admit you have an addiction or mental illness because you are tired of living life without the proper medication and that you are tired of the same ole same ole—stigma and shame.

Mary/Pumpkin would accept that God did not design her to live a life of bondage and defeat.

Here at the detox psych ward, she would learn every addiction and mental illness was different.

In the group settings, Mary/Pumpkin would learn that people who are trapped in addiction had no peace in their life. Most group topics always ended with the patients saying nothing they found gave them peace until they came to the detox ward.

They would say neither money, sex, nor drugs gave them peace they needed. In the group session, she would learn to accept herself where she was in her addiction and to accept she was going to need help from her treatment plan, for her body was going to go through a physical and mental change now that she was five days clean.

The basic principle for the addict trapped by any form of addiction is asking for help and to be willing to go through the experience and steps needed to reach their goal for recovery.

For most addicts, not accepting you have a problem keeps you in the chains of addiction.

There is help out there for any addict trapped in a life of addiction. There is help, hope, and people who share a common bond. There are survivors of addiction, and there are survivors who live functioning lives with co-occurring disorders.

In group sessions, Mary/Pumpkin had to learn people will talk about you no matter if you are doing well and they will talk about you if you are doing badly. Unhappy people like to cause confusion to keep the focus off them so they will talk about people to create the illusion they have power over you. See, those are the ones who want to get you back in the dungeon.

Unhappy people want to keep happy people down. Mary/Pumpkin had to get her mind clear; it was almost time to leave the safety of the detox ward, for Mary/Pumpkin started realizing the devil and his demons were waiting for her in *The City*.

For the first time since arriving at the detox ward, Mary/Pumpkin had not cried for at least three days. For her that was progress.

One day after group, one of the patients came to Mary/Pumpkin and asked if he could draw a picture of her.

Mary/Pumpkin was apprehensive because this patient liked to intimidate many of the patients. He had the appearance of the wrestler on World Wrestling named Andre the Giant. Man, you should have seen him—he looked like he was ready to beat up anyone that he didn't like! Yet he liked Mary/Pumpkin—maybe it was the fact she whispered in his ear that she was not afraid of him.

With nothing to fear, she said yes. They both went into the TV room and there he drew her picture. When he was finished he would tell Mary/Pumpkin to keep this picture and never forget she was a survivor and God had great work for her to do.

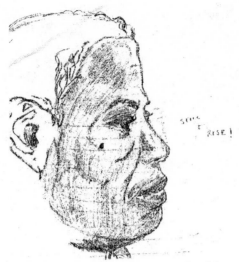

Mary/Pumpkin was so proud of her picture she would show it to the staff and anyone that would look at it. For on the picture he wrote *Still I Rise*, as if God used His picture to give Mary/Pumpkin more insight to the unseen purpose of her life.

One of the nurses on duty asked her, "Mary/Pumpkin, what did you do for this patient to engage with you with no problems?"

"I treated him like I wanted to be treated, not as a patient but a human."

You should have seen the nurse's face. Every person with mental health disorders, addiction, or suicide has a story. The real problem with people with co-occurring disorders is that *no one is listening*.

Exhausted, Mary/Pumpkin retired to her room. Realizing she was approaching her time for discharge, Mary/Pumpkin looked at herself in the mirror and said her most powerful words: "I will not leave the detox psych ward as Mary/Pumpkin; my name is Mary and I am happy to be back. Thank you, Jesus Christ, for sending me to the detox psych ward, for this place has changed my life forever."

Yet for Mary the true test of recovery was about to happen now that she was leaving her safety zone.

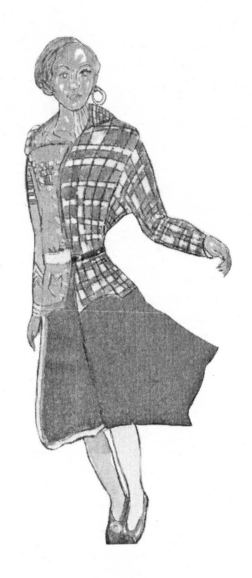

Chapter 7

Putting It All Together Again

Has there ever been a time in your life when you forgot who you were? Or where you were? Or who you belong to?

Time had passed and Mary forgot who she was. No longer able to run from herself, she was ready to accept the slogan *Change I must or die I will* attitude. Putting it all together again is the beginning for the addict to admit their wrong and work with professional rehabilitation programs to reach the truth.

The detox psych ward gave her the tools to start putting it together. But putting it *all* together would take courage and support to achieve this new way of living.

No addict can put it together alone, whether it's at a rehab or an out- or in-patient psychiatric ward, or group sessions or one-on-one therapy. One person cannot do it alone.

Sure, some don't need AA or NA and some don't need a therapist or the need to attend church. But every recovery person had to find a source to cope and deal with life on life's terms.

The recovery addict must have some form of a recovery program or discipline to stop living with their addictive behavior.

For Mary, a recovery program would mean working with a strong-minded person to help her weak-minded behavioral without judgment. For Mary, she had to learn how to fight obstacles when coming to the fork in the road, and how to reach and achieve personal goals, even if she relapsed.

For any person who may not be aware, the purposes of recovery programs are to help the addict learn important truths about who they are with knowledge to know what to do if they relapse. No addict in recovery will achieve success from the beginning. It's a process.

Although Mary went to several rehab programs, all she kept hearing was her grandma's voice saying, "You must know God for yourself, and always be prepared when trouble happens that you must believe and know prayer works."

For Mary to reach success in her recovery, she had to have the spirit of God. For anyone who believes the enemy is going to let you out of a life of addiction, depression, and despair without a fight, you are setting yourself up for failure.

Mary faced challenges that most addicts in recovery face every day: learning how to say no to something that is easier said than done.

Putting it all together again meant she had to learn to work with the right prescription medication for depression. It was only her prescription medication that would give her a fighting chance with the drugs. She had to start telling herself every day to stay focused and to stay committed to whatever she said she was going to do after she left the detox center.

In staying focused, Mary created a three-step survival plan for herself to create discipline and balance not to use drugs while living in *The City*.

1. *Her purpose:* find a therapist
2. *Her plan:* move from *The City*
3. *Her goal:* find rehabilitation day programs to attend

Mary knew it was time to stop compromising principle and allowing her addiction to keep her in despair. She knew it was time to start producing a life of maturity to live in recovery and not die in her co-occurring disorder.

For Mary, this new way of thinking seemed overwhelming, for living in *The City*, drugs were at her front door. Recovery for Mary would mean a life alone until she became strong enough to face those people, places, and situations, and her family. Her most important challenge: She had to accept she was not going to allow her family to put her down about her addiction.

Mary remembered in a group session how one of the patients said he had been clean for a week and his family got on his nerves so bad all he wanted to do was escape by drinking and drugging. Mary knew it could happen so she had to decide between loneliness or death.

See, Mary had to learn the benefits of life without her drugs. She had to learn what benefits are there to being alone.

Being alone brought Mary peace of mind to look at life from a different prospective. She would get clarity why she went through the fires of addiction and why her life from a child to an adult was broken into many pieces. Being alone and having peace of mind made her appreciate her life's journey. Mary would come to terms that through it all, she knew Jesus Christ loved her and He would never put more on her than she could bear.

Putting it all together again means you can look in the mirror and see a new person and forgive yourself by understanding yes I made mistakes but I will not allow my mistakes of the past to control my future.

One day Mary was looking in the mirror she remembered all the times she cried and how she never liked to see her reflections of pain and hurt from her addiction. Yet on this day she smiled and laughed. For the first time she was happy with what she seen. There was no pain and there was no tears falling from her face. Then she looked again and knew there was no more Pumpkin. Pumpkin was gone.

The difference for Mary: She did not have to use drugs to win this journey. Mary is a new creature and recovery is her friend. Mary will be the first to tell you recovery has not been easy. She knew there would be times she would fall. It's all a part of recovery. Yet she did not give up! When she felt overwhelmed, she would find a meeting and when she felt suicidal she checked herself into a psych ward.

If you ask Mary what are the keys to success in recovery, she would tell anyone that success is getting information with the mental or behavioral department in your city, state, or town until you get the professional help you need.

No matter how often the recovering addict falls down, don't give up and never give in. Mary will always be an addict; she has only learned sometimes harm reduction can give you a fighting chance until you totally allow a Higher Power to fix it.

Putting It All Together Again means for the addict in recovery, it is important to understand *relapse will happen, just don't use it as an excuse to play the addiction game by fooling yourself.*

The road to recovery has many ups and downs. For any addict with an addiction, the best thing to remember is that help is out there; *never fear change; it's for the better not the bitter!* While you are seeking help for your addiction or mental health disorder, always put on your Helmet of Salvation, with your Breast Plate of Righteousness, along with your Shield of Faith, and your Sword of Victory!

Mary had to always keep in mind all things are possible to them that believe and Mary had to accept her co-occurring disorders will be her lifelong journey. However, she could live a normal life as long as she faced life on life terms by identifying who and what are her Judas Iscariots.

Mary would say your Judas Iscariot could be your family, friends, children, relationship, and even your job—anything that causes you to relapse, for the devil will use people, places, situations, and family to create the way for you to fail and fall.

For whosoever understands this parable: must believe everything has a season, even when you are going through, God favors you! The test and trails that come in your life are to make you strong when you are lost; all praises go to our God, for the battle is not yours when you fall down. Just get back up and try it again. Don't give up! Let go and Let God. He might not come when you want Him, but He is an on time God. Whatever it is maybe God is trying to tell you something: that the change will come and you will be free. He is able, how great is God's mercy He will not put more on you than you can bare: so don't worry; the storm is over for God's timing is not yours.

Just think of all the challenges and changes Mary went through to get to her purpose to share the message of hope through her memoirs.

Her faith and relationship with her Higher Power gave her understanding that all things used for negative such as her secret pains, hurt, and despair, God is going to use for positive to help someone in the struggle with co-occurring disorders.

From her personal relationship with her Savior, Mary gained peace through confusion and she received unconditional love through sorrow.

Mary has accepted the greatest lesson of all— that recovery is an every second, every minute, every hour, every day process…and it is *possible.*

Smiling and being grateful for her life, Mary would open her Bible and read a scripture that would be a foundation, testimony, and victory to her life as an addict.

Psalms 30

I will exalt thee. O Lord for you have lifted me up
and did not let my enemies rejoices over me.

O Lord my God, I called to you for help and you
healed me.

O Lord you have brought my soul from the grave
and have kept me alive that I did not go down into
the pit.

Sing unto the Lord, O ye saints of his and give
thanks at the remembrance of his holiness

For his anger last but a moment: in his favor is life

Weeping may endure for a night but joy cometh in
the morning.

And in my prosperity I said, I shall never be moved.

O Lord when you favored me you made my
mountain stand firm but when you hid your face I
was trouble.

To you, O Lord, I called, I cried for mercy.

What profit us there in my blood when I go down
into the pit?
Will the dust praise you? Will it proclaim your
faithfulness?

Hear O Lord and have mercy upon me: Lord, be my helper.

Thou have turned my mourning into dancing: thou hast put off my sackcloth and girded me with gladness:

To the end that my heart may sing praises to you, and not be silent.

O Lord my God, I will give you thanks for ever.

Amen

To those who understand my story and
to those who may judge my story…
I encourage all to be strong and
courageous.

Seek and find your own personal
scripture or prayer and include yourself as if
you and your God of understanding are in
conversation.

Let your personal scripture or prayer be
your source for strength and power
when life shows up.

The End

Memoirs Of An Addict:
Fact or Fiction

Workbook

Facts to Discover & Points to Ponder

This portion of the book contains {**Facts to Discover & Points to Ponder**} a self-paced educational workbook that can be used for personal and or group discussions.

Each section of the workbook will enlighten, educate and empower you with a general perspective of Co-Occurring Disorders that includes; writing exercises, fill-in-the-blanks; open ended questions and information that can be used for personal and critical thinking.

The beauty of this workbook there is no timeframe or order as to when it is completed.

DISCLAIMER:

When reading and participating with this workbook
if you feel any of the issues herein apply to you
personally, you are encouraged to seek an assessment
from a qualified Behavioral Health Professional.

Did you know?

The National Institute for Mental Health states: Personality disorders are mental disorders characterized by enduring, inflexible, and maladaptive personality traits that deviate markedly from cultural expectations, pervade a broad range of situations, and are either a source of subjective distress or a cause of significant impairment in social, occupational, or other functioning. In general, they are difficult both to diagnose and to treat. People with borderline personality disorder and those with narcissistic personality disorder both may have a tendency to angry outbursts and may be hindered in forming interpersonal relationships because they often exploit, idealize, or devalue others. More than one personality disorder can exist in the same person although individuals with a personality disorder can function in day-to-day life, they are hampered both emotionally and psychologically by the maladaptive nature of their disorder, and their chances of forming good relationships and fulfilling their potentialities are poor. In spite of their problems, these patients refuse to acknowledge that anything is wrong and insist that it is the rest of the world that is out of step. Very often their behavior is extremely annoying to those around them. Personality disorders result from unresolved conflicts, often dating back to childhood. To alleviate the anxiety and depression that accompany these conflicts, the ego uses defense mechanisms. Although defense mechanisms are not pathological in themselves, they become maladaptive in individuals with personality disorders. THE WELL-ADJUSTED PERSONALITY, A well-adjusted individual is one who adapts to surroundings. If adaptation is not possible, the individual makes realistic efforts to change the situation, using personal talents and abilities constructively and successfully. The well-adjusted person is realistic and able to face facts whether they are pleasant or unpleasant, and deals with them instead of merely worrying about them or denying them. Well-adjusted mature persons are independent. They form reasoned opinions and then act on them. They seek a reasonable amount of information and advice before making a decision, and once the decision is made, they are willing to face the consequences of it. They do not try to force others to make decisions for them. An ability to love others is typical of the well-adjusted individual. In addition, the mature well-adjusted person is also able to enjoy receiving love and affection and can accept a reasonable dependence on others. The symptoms of a personality disorder may occur as mental disorder.[1]

---

[1] NIMH National Institute of Mental Health

Affect or Effect

The IMPORTANCE of understanding the four levels of the physical health, mental health, spiritual health and emotional health.

Define the words below

Then write a sentence explaining the similarities and or dissimilarities of the physical, mental, emotional, and spiritual health and how each affects or effects the body with addiction and mental health disorders.

Physical

Mental

Spiritual

Emotional

Art therapy

Where do you hurt and why?

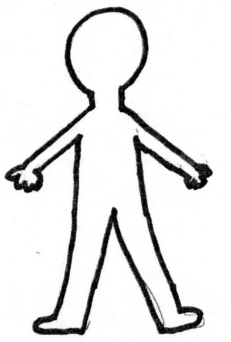

Draw your emotions with colors, pictures or
symbols to describe how you feel.

136

Did you know some individuals with Co-Occurring Disorders **do not address** substance use and mental health disorders singularly or collectively because they do not believe it is **relevant** to their problems?

From the list of Mental Health Disorders below write a sentence how each *Disorder* is affected with an Addiction Disorder.

- **Major Depressive disorder:**

- **Anxiety**

- **Schizophrenia:**

- **Schizoaffective Disorder:**

- **PSTD:**

- **Bipolar I, Disorders:**

- **Bipolar II, Disorders:**

- **Personality Disorder:**

- Obsessive Compulsive Disorder:

- Caffeine Related Disorder:

- Cannabis Dependence Disorder:

- Binge Eating Disorder:

- Bibliomania Disorder:

- Narcissistic Disorder:

- Bereavement:

- Sexual disorders

- Sleep disorders

Facts to Discover & Points to Ponder

What are Co-Occurring Disorders?

_____

_____

_____

_____

_____

_____

_____

_____

_____

_____

_____

_____

_____

_____

_____

_____

Write the definition for the following words and their correlation to addiction.

Dopamine_____

_____
_____
_____
_____
_____

Endorphins_____

_____
_____
_____
_____
_____
_____
_____

Serotonin_____

_____
_____
_____
_____
_____
_____

Facts to Discover & Points to Ponder

What is your definition of the word **addict?**

What is the dictionary definition of the word **addict?**

Now compare your answers

Write and explain the effects each has on the brain and body.

Dopamine_____

_____
_____
_____
_____
_____

Endorphins_____

_____
_____
_____
_____
_____
_____

Serotonin_____

_____
_____
_____
_____
_____
_____

What is a habit?

_____
_____
_____
_____
_____
_____
_____
_____
_____
_____
_____
_____
_____
_____
_____

143

What is your definition of the word **addiction**?

What is the dictionary definition of the word **addiction**?

Now compare your answers

Facts to Discover & Points to Ponder

Let's Talk…Is addiction and abuse the same?

_____

_____

_____

_____

_____

_____

_____

_____

_____

_____

_____

_____

_____

_____

_____

_____

_____

_____

_____

_____

Write the definition for the following words. Then describe the similarities and dissimilarities of the behavioral characteristics.

Obsessive-

_____

_____

_____

_____

Compulsive-

_____

_____

_____

_____

Addictive-

_____

_____

_____

_____

146

Facts to Discover & Points to Ponder

Write the definition for the following words?

Psychiatrist_____

_____

_____

Psychologist_____

_____

_____

Counselor_____

_____

_____

Social
worker_____

_____

_____

Therapist_____

_____

_____

Let's talk…Do you know who you are?

Facts to Discover & Points to Ponder

Write 5 positive things about yourself

1.

2.

3.

4.

5.

Do you think most addictions start with having a dysfunctional family?

_____
_____
_____
_____
_____
_____
_____
_____
_____
_____
_____
_____
_____
_____
_____
_____
_____
_____
_____
_____

What is your definition of the word **normal**?

What does behavioral health and the dictionary's definition of the word **normal** represents?

Now compare your answers.

Cognitive Behavioral Therapy

Write the definition for (CBT). Then explain if **any** what the benefits are.

_____

_____

_____

_____

_____

_____

_____

_____

_____

_____

_____

_____

_____

_____

_____

_____

_____

_____

Write and explain the dictionary's definition for
the follow words

CRAZY

_____
_____
_____
_____
_____
_____
_____
_____

INSANE

_____
_____
_____
_____
_____
_____
_____
_____
_____
_____

Let's talk…What is the difference between a consumer of behavioral health verses a client of behavioral health?

_____

_____

_____

_____

_____

_____

_____

_____

_____

_____

_____

_____

_____

_____

The POSTIVE Alphabets

Create a word for each letter that describes a positive emotion.

A.

B.

C.

D.

E.

F.

G.

H.

I.

J.

K.

L.

M.

N.

O.

P.

Q.

R.

S.

T.

U.

V.

W.

X.

Y.

Z.

Describe the meaning of the following words?

Mental Health
disorders_____

_____
_____
_____

Substance abuse
disorders_____

_____
_____
_____

Suicidal
ideations_____

_____
_____
_____
_____
_____

Let's Talk...What is Autonomy? Now explain what is Perception in behavioral health?

_____

_____

_____

_____

_____

_____

_____

_____

_____

_____

_____

_____

_____

_____

_____

_____

_____

_____

_____

What does Continuity of Care mean?

_____

_____

_____

_____

_____

_____

_____

_____

_____

_____

_____

_____

_____

_____

_____

_____

_____

_____

_____

_____

What are the 5 Stages of Change in recovery?

Can you name them all?

1.

2.

3.

4.

5.

Define the following words

Relapse

_____

_____

_____

_____

_____

_____

Decompensation

_____

_____

_____

_____

_____

_____

_____

What HOPE Looks Like

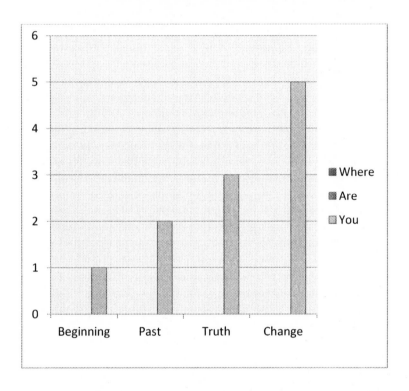

Mary/Pumpkin's Life Chart

The Beginning	Identifying
The Past	Understanding
The Truth	Accepting
The Change	Believing

Create a short story about yourself applying the examples below.

THE
BEGINNING_____
_____
_____

THE
PAST_____
_____
_____

THE
TRUTH_____
_____
_____

THE
CHANGE_____
_____
_____

What is the purpose of Motivational Interviewing?

Should a person always tell the TRUTH?

_____

_____

_____

_____

_____

_____

_____

_____

_____

_____

_____

_____

_____

_____

_____

_____

_____

_____

_____

_____

_____

Mary/Pumpkin's personal questions of...

Truth or Deceit

Is my life the way it is because of others?

Am I happy with myself as a person?

Do I accept where I am in my life?

Does my co-occurring disorder play a part of all my decisions?

What must I do to help myself to improve and change?

Is there ever a right TIME to tell a lie? Explain

_____

_____

_____

_____

_____

_____

_____

_____

_____

_____

_____

_____

_____

_____

_____

_____

_____

_____

_____

_____

_____

What is a Paradigm Shift?

Create and draw your Family Tree

Addiction, Mental Health and Incarceration

Do they go together?

_____
_____
_____
_____
_____
_____
_____
_____
_____
_____
_____
_____
_____
_____
_____
_____
_____
_____
_____

169

Stress Management

1. What is stress management?

2. How does stress affect the body?

3. How should a person handle stressful situations?

_____
_____
_____
_____
_____
_____
_____
_____
_____
_____
_____
_____
_____
_____
_____
_____
_____
_____
_____

Abuse, rejection, loneliness and neglect can be signs of trauma.

Can you name any other signs that might indicate a person has experienced trauma?

_____

_____

_____

_____

_____

_____

_____

_____

_____

_____

_____

_____

_____

_____

_____

_____

_____

_____

_____

_____

Facts to Discover & Points to Ponder

What does the term escapism means?

_____

_____

_____

_____

_____

_____

_____

_____

_____

_____

_____

_____

_____

_____

_____

_____

_____

_____

_____

_____

_____

What is the difference between empathy and sympathy?

_____

_____

_____

_____

_____

_____

_____

_____

_____

_____

_____

_____

_____

_____

_____

_____

_____

_____

What is **your** definition of the following words below?

Reality_____
_____
_____

Fantasy_____
_____
_____

Paranoia_____
_____
_____

How does the dictionary define these words?

Facts to Discover & Points to Ponder

In order for Mary/Pumpkin to move forward in her recovery she had to gain an understanding that there are different hallucinations such as:

Tactile	Touch
Olfactory	Smell
Auditory	Hear
Visual	See
Gustatory	Taste

Most importantly she had to gain understanding when her hallucinations were real or not.

What are hallucinations?

_____

_____

_____

_____

_____

_____

_____

_____

_____

_____

_____

_____

_____

_____

_____

_____

_____

_____

_____

_____

Let's Talk… Anxiety and Addiction, how do they interact with each other?

_____

_____

_____

_____

_____

_____

_____

_____

_____

_____

_____

_____

_____

_____

_____

_____

_____

_____

_____

_____

How many celebrities can you name that **have died** from addiction and or mental health disorders?

AIDS verses HIV

What is HIV?

_____

_____

_____

How does it affect the body?

What is AIDS?

_____

_____

_____

How does it affect the body?

What Is The DIFFERENCE?

_____

_____

_____

How can one get the disease?

179

How many celebrities have exhibited successful recovery from addiction and or mental health disorders?

Let's talk...Integrity

How does integrity affect a person's life with or without an addiction and or mental health

co-occurring disorders?

Please Don't!

When you come to the fork in the road ONLY YOU CAN   decide which way to go.

The struggle between good and bad is not to be an easy choice

It is a FREE WILL decision.

**Before you make up your mind to judge me...
Please Don't!**

You need to walk in my shoes and come to an understand

Of

FAITH and POWER

In something greater than ourselves

- Memoirs Rhonda Johnson

2013

What is rejection?

_____
_____
_____
_____
_____
_____
_____
_____
_____
_____
_____
_____
_____
_____
_____
_____
_____
_____
_____

Can a person with a mental health disorder live a normal life?

_____

_____

_____

_____

_____

_____

_____

_____

_____

_____

_____

_____

_____

_____

_____

_____

_____

_____

_____

_____

Facts to Discover & Points to Ponder

What does recovery mean to you?

_____

_____

_____

_____

_____

_____

_____

_____

_____

_____

_____

_____

_____

_____

_____

_____

_____

_____

_____

_____

What is your definition of the word **triggers**?

What is the dictionary definition of the word **triggers**?

Do you know if you have any triggers?

Now compare your answers

Facts to Discover & Points to Ponder

Trigger signs come in many forms such as:

- Depression

- Anger

- Boredom

- Disappointment

- Financial problems

Can you name any others triggers that can affect a person with co-occurring disorders?

What is Intervention?

_____

_____

_____

_____

_____

_____

_____

_____

_____

_____

_____

_____

_____

_____

_____

_____

_____

_____

_____

When an addict is in recovery SHOULD their family members participate in their recovery program?

Anger Management

What is Anger Management?

_____

_____

_____

_____

_____

_____

_____

What are some positive tools one can use to address anger issues?

_____

_____

_____

_____

_____

_____

Coping Skills

Name some COPING SKILLS a person can or should use when being tempted in their addiction, mental health disorder and or co-occurring disorders?

Let's talk...Can a person move forward with
unresolved issues of abuse and or addictions?

_____

_____

_____

_____

_____

_____

_____

_____

_____

_____

_____

_____

_____

_____

_____

_____

_____

_____

The Negative Alphabets

Create a word for each letter that describes a negative emotion.

A.	N.
B.	O.
C.	P.
D.	Q.
E.	R.
F.	S.
G.	T.
H.	U.
I.	V.
J.	W.
K.	X.
L.	Y.
M.	Z.

Let's talk…How does one reach out for HELP?

_____

_____

_____

_____

_____

_____

_____

_____

_____

_____

_____

_____

_____

_____

_____

_____

_____

_____

_____

_____

Do you think self-esteem plays a factor in addiction?

_____

_____

_____

_____

_____

_____

_____

_____

_____

_____

_____

_____

_____

_____

_____

_____

_____

_____

_____

_____

What are some **SIGNS** an addiction is out of control?

_____

_____

_____

_____

_____

_____

_____

_____

_____

_____

_____

_____

_____

_____

_____

_____

_____

_____

What is the **difference** between Recovery Rehabilitation Centers verses Mental Health Psychiatric Ward?

_____

_____

_____

_____

_____

_____

_____

_____

_____

_____

_____

_____

_____

_____

_____

_____

_____

_____

_____

_____

_____

_____

Name **some reasons** why a person may have an addiction.

_____

_____

_____

_____

_____

_____

_____

_____

_____

_____

_____

_____

_____

_____

_____

_____

_____

_____

What is Integrative Care Treatment?

_____

_____

_____

_____

_____

_____

_____

_____

_____

_____

_____

_____

_____

_____

_____

_____

_____

_____

_____

_____

_____

_____

_____

199

Create a personal BILL OF RIGHTS according to your own **morals, beliefs, ethics** and **judgments.**

Google Bill of Rights in Recovery

_____

_____

_____

_____

_____

_____

_____

_____

_____

_____

_____

_____

_____

_____

_____

_____

Write 5 things you would like to accomplish in your life.

1.

2.

3.

4.

5.

Now chose 3 from the 5 you believe can be manifested into existence.

1.

2.

3.

Rethink your thinking watch the movie

A Beautiful Mind

What does Co-Morbidity mean?

_____

_____

_____

_____

_____

_____

_____

_____

_____

_____

_____

_____

_____

_____

_____

_____

_____

_____

_____

_____

_____

What does Stages of TREATMENT in behavioral health mean? Can you name them?

Facts to Discover & Points to Ponder

What is Harm Reduction?

_____

_____

_____

_____

_____

_____

_____

_____

_____

_____

_____

_____

_____

_____

_____

_____

_____

_____

_____

_____

The term "Self-Medicate"

What do you think it means?

_____

_____

_____

_____

_____

_____

_____

_____

_____

_____

_____

_____

_____

_____

_____

_____

_____

_____

_____

_____

Do you agree or dis-agree that addiction and mental health disorders are both chemical imbalances of the brain?

_____

_____

_____

_____

_____

_____

_____

_____

_____

_____

_____

_____

_____

_____

_____

_____

_____

Name some **myths** concerning addiction and mental
health disorders

_____

_____

_____

_____

_____

_____

_____

_____

_____

_____

_____

_____

_____

_____

_____

_____

_____

_____

_____

_____

How many words can you make from the word
RECOVERY?

What is your definition of the word **recovery**?

What is the dictionary definition of the word **recovery**?

Now compare your answers.

Facts to Discover & Points to Ponder

Let's Talk... What are your views, thoughts and theories regarding tolerance as related to co-occurring disorders?

_____

_____

_____

_____

_____

_____

_____

_____

_____

_____

_____

_____

_____

_____

_____

_____

_____

How many movies can you name that were based on addiction and or mental health disorders?

_____

_____

_____

_____

_____

_____

_____

_____

_____

_____

_____

_____

_____

_____

_____

_____

_____

_____

_____

Facts to Discover & Points to Ponder

Briefly write your thoughts, ideas, dreams, goals and future achievements **you desire to have in place** to move to the next level in your life?

_____

_____

_____

_____

_____

_____

_____

_____

_____

_____

_____

_____

_____

_____

_____

_____

_____

_____

_____

Words of Wisdom -Mr. Mario Richardson 2012

Write a poem about LOVE.

_____

_____

_____

_____

_____

_____

_____

_____

_____

_____

_____

_____

_____

_____

_____

_____

_____

Other than a person dealing with the shame and the stigma of co-occurring disorders name some reasons that keep so many people from reaching out for help?

Mary/Pumpkin created a creed for survival. What is the definition of the word CREED?

_____

_____

_____

Create your own CREED for the following:

People:

_____

_____

_____

_____

Places:

_____

_____

_____

_____

Things:

_____

_____

_____

216

How can one help someone who is reaching out for help and looking for answers of hope and encouragement?

_____

_____

_____

_____

_____

_____

_____

_____

_____

_____

_____

_____

_____

_____

_____

_____

_____

With all that has been said and done, what is truly the meaning of life?

_____

_____

_____

_____

_____

_____

_____

_____

_____

_____

_____

_____

_____

_____

_____

_____

_____

_____

_____

_____

Facts to Discover & Points to Ponder

Can an addict ever be free?

_____

_____

_____

_____

_____

_____

_____

_____

_____

_____

_____

_____

_____

_____

_____

_____

Facts to Discover & Points to Ponder

Fill in the blanks

I was once _____

But now I _____

I was _____

But now I can _____

Personal Notes

Personal Notes

Personal Notes

Personal Notes

Personal Notes

Personal Notes

Personal Notes

Personal Notes

Personal Notes

Personal Notes

Personal Notes

Personal Notes

Personal Notes

Personal Notes

Where to seek HELP and TREATMENT

Below is a list of some organizations with Help- lines and email addresses that can point you in the right direction when seeking answers concerning behavioral health disorders.

Anyone that feels they are in **CRISIS DIAL 911**

National Suicide Prevention Lifeline
www.suicidepreventionlife.org **1-800 273.8255**

NIMH: National Institute of Mental Health
www.nimh.gov

SAMHSA: Substance Abuse and Mental Health Services Administration www.samhsa.gov

NAMI: National Alliance on Mental Health
www.nami.org

Veterans Crisis line 1-800 273-8255
www.veteranscrisisline.net

Boys Town National Hotline 1-800 448-3000

www.boystown.org/hotline

GLBT National Help Center 1-888 843-4564

www.glbtnationalhelpcenter.org

Problem Gambling Helpline 1-800 426-2537
www.ncpgambling.org

Sex Addiction Hotline 1-800 477-8191

www.saa-recovery.org

The Truth about Drugs
www.drugfreeworld.org

National Council for Behavioral Health
www.thenationalcouncil.org

Mental Health America MHA
www.mentalhealthamerica.net

CCUSA: Catholic Charities USA
www.catholiccharitiesusa.org

AA Alcoholics Anonymous www.aa.org

NA Narcotics Anonymous www.na.org

Salvation Army www.salvationarmy.org

Depression and Bipolar Support Alliance
www.dbsalliance.org

Get Smart About Drug

www.getsmartaboutdrug.com

Access Helpline/dbh Washington, D.C.

1-888 793-4357
www.dbh.D.C.gov/services/access-helpline.com

Suicide Hotline 1-800 suicide

Contact your Department of Behavioral Health for mobile crisis, children, mental health, or military assistance in your city, town or state.

YOU ARE NOT ALONE, HELP IS OUT THERE!

Let's Talk...

People are asking questions and they are reaching out for answers

Share your stories on suicide, addiction and or mental health disorders.

Then share your WISDOM of

Hope, Recovery and Survival

with the

MEMOIRS INFORMER

Together we can **educate** and **advocate** for change!

For submission requirements email

www.mrjohnson2165@Outlook.com

ACKNOWLEDGEMENTS

Giving HONOR, GLORY and THANKS to the Almighty God Jesus the Christ who provided me with the courage, vision, strength and love to carry the message of HOPE to the next level.

To the late Nathaniel and Patricia Johnson the greatest parents this side of earth. Thank you mommy and daddy for always being examples what makes a family, and what family love is made of. Not only were you sent from God, you truly demonstrated that love and marriage can work. Thank you for your presence and spirit that kept encouraging me that I could complete this book. I miss and love you so much.

To the late Virginia Simms my Big Mama, a true woman of God. Thank you for always wiping my tears and holding my hands. Big Mama your presence is missed by many. Thank you for introducing me to Jesus Christ to learn and understand the POWER within me. I am forever grateful.

To the late CoReda Jones, thank you God's Angel for introducing me to fasting, praying and carrying all concerns to the mirror to talk to Jesus and tell Him about all my struggles.

To Triple J my children Jeffrey, Jamar and Jasmine plus 1 Neysa you all are my life. Thank you for always loving your mother and ALWAYS being there for me through the good and not so good times. Thank you for your unconditional love. It was your love why I never gave up. I love you all {Ron-Ron}

To Ashley B. Johnson Don't Give Up on your dreams of being a #1 vocal artist and to Joseph {Bam -Bam} Bragg.   I love you both.

To GiGi girls Hailey Isabella {Tink-Tink} and Abigail Rose {Wink-Wink} because of you two I now understand the meaning of life. Hugs and Kisses to **all** my future Grandbabies that are on the way.

To Antonio Sr., Joseph Sr., Vakisa, all my aunts, all my uncles, all my cousins, all my nieces, all my nephews, Neysa Sr., Brandi, my in-laws and close and best friends, I love you **ALL!**

Thank you to my friend Grady T. for pointing me back to who I was a **WINNER.** Thank you for giving me my everyday talk and encouragement to just do something positive with my life when all I could see was darkness.

To all the Warriors and Soldiers God placed in my life while I was in my addiction and mental health state of mind, thank you **all** for always making sure I was safe in Ivy City, 7th Street, Trinidad and Florida Ave.

To my Godmother Barbara Jean and God Sister Channy, I thank God for allowing me to meet your family so I could have an extended family that loved Mary/Rhonda for me. I love you all so much!

Giving honor to **All** my Church Pastors, the late Dr. Fernette Nichols-*God's Universal Kingdom*, Bishop Michael and Sheila Kelsey- *New Samaritan Baptist Church* and my awesome Pastor Patrick J. Walker Sr., First Lady Priscella Walker and my church family - *The New Macedonia Baptist Church*. Thank you **All** for your spiritual leadership. I am truly Blessed.

Many thanks to Mr. Stephen Baron, The Director of Department of Behavioral Health, Washington, D.C., Mrs.Vivi Smith, Director of the Office of Consumer and Family Affairs, Adrienne Lightfoot, CPS, Rossine Minard, CPS and Mrs. Angele Moss-Baker MA, LPC, D.C.MHS Co-Occurring Disorders Training Coordinator.

Thank you to Catholic Charities, Archdiocese of Washington, D.C., Msgr. John Enzler, President and CEO, Director Denise Capaci, Adult & Children Clinical Services, Karen Ostlie, Dr. Irvin Barnes, and Sharon Guevara for the opportunity to work as a Certified Peer Specialist at Anchor Mental Health {ACT} Assertive Community Treatment Team. Most importantly thank you to **All my co-workers** and the staff in the building you are the *BEST*.

Thank you to the Staff of Byte Back Computer Program, Washington, D.C., for the skills, the computer and internet service to begin my life's journey.

To the Staff at the Martin Luther King Jr. Library Washington, D.C., I am forever grateful for the computer classes, events and knowledge the library provides. Thank you to Mr. Michael Price and Ms. Desiré P. Grogan.

To Yousef Tarrah, of Copy Rite Printing & Imaging Washington, D.C. Wow! Yousef, your company is AWESOME! Thank you for working with me over a year with making sure my book cover was the way I envisioned it to be. I appreciate your professionalism. You are the best!

To Mr. Leon Odoms, thank you for making sure Mary/Pumpkin was everything I wanted her to be. She is beautiful because of your art work. I wish you much SUCCESS!

Thank you to my book doctor Kristen of Kristen House Manuscript Editing Corrects Service for being the BEST editor. Thank you for your prompt service and responding to all my concerns. Your professional editing company truly offers high-quality work. I highly recommend your services.

To JoMar Wilson RN, BSN, Thank you for agreeing to edit my workbook with your medical expertise. JoMar you are more than my editor you are my friend. Thank you for your 39 years of professional service in the health field of medicine. Love you girl!

Thank you Dr. Tiffany N. Johnson-Largent, Ph.D., RD, LN, LD, for being my first source of inspiration as well as my first proof reader. It was your encouragements that inspire me I could write this book and make a difference.

Thank you to the staff of Trinity Square Behavioral Health Washington Hospital Center. Thank you Dr. Clay Sounder and Mr. Corey Beauford for observing when I was at the lowest point in my life you both gave me hope and made SURE that I received the correct help and treatment.

To Laura B. my therapist thank you for allowing me to walk through the dark doors of sadness and encouraging me that there was a way out of the black hole of depression called HOPE, yes I was never a TROUBLE MAKER just a TRUTH SAYER. Lo! I love you Laura

To Mrs. Porter my therapist thank you for creating an environment for me to accept my destiny and to welcome who I am by understanding my purpose in a Higher Power. Thank you for letting me see through our sessions I am more than what I was and to stop blaming and start accepting. I am forever grateful.

To Bernice Brown, Mary J, Tammy, Angie, Anthony, Tara, Mr. Mario Richardson, TEAM Clerical, **ALL my friends that are to many to name,** Ms. Vanessa the Office Assistant, Ms. Irish, **the ENTIRE STAFF** *and* Dr. Yvonne B. Ali, President of PSI Washington D.C. Rehabilitation Day Program, THANK YOU ALL for your everyday support, friendship, my birthday party, love, and encouragement, that having a mental disorder was not the end of the world.

ABOUT THE AUTHOR

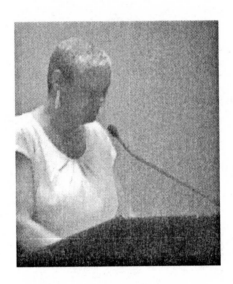

M/R Johnson was born and raised in the Nation's Capital Washington D.C. She is a graduate from the Washington, D.C. Department of Behavioral Health Co-Occurring Clinical Competence Course and the Office of Consumers and Family Affairs Certified Peer Specialist Certification Program.

Compelled by society's misunderstanding of Co-Occurring Disorders, M/R Johnson offers insight from a dynamic perspective, drawing from her personal lived experiences, clinical education and professional work background on an Assertive Community Treatment Team. M/R Johnson believes her time has come, and that no matter what challenges a person encounters in this road to life, "All things are possible with FAITH in God!"

For Media and Public Speaking Inquiries
Email: mrjohnson2165 @ Outlook.com

DON'T GIVE UP!

MEMOIRS OF AN ADDICT: FACT OR FICTION
{THEME SONG} COPYRIGHT © 2013

Don't Give Up! HE will help you through anything

Don't Give Up! The pain will end

Don't Give Up!

Your sorrow will descend; HE will help you through, HE will help you move. If you want to change, you got to rearrange your life and give it to GOD he will work it out.

So Don't Give Up!

Now if you are down and you need help.

HE will pick you up,

HE will turn you around. HE will place you on better ground and give you what you need!

So go forward, and if you got a problem, you should give it to GOD and HE will work it out.

HE has a journey for you; because

HE is talking to you

Now if you are listening HE is saying

Don't Give Up!

Don't Give Up! So Don't Give Up! Just Don't You Give Up!

Remember Don't Give Up On God!

I STAND AT THE DOOR AND KNOCK

www. Memoirs Of 2165.Com